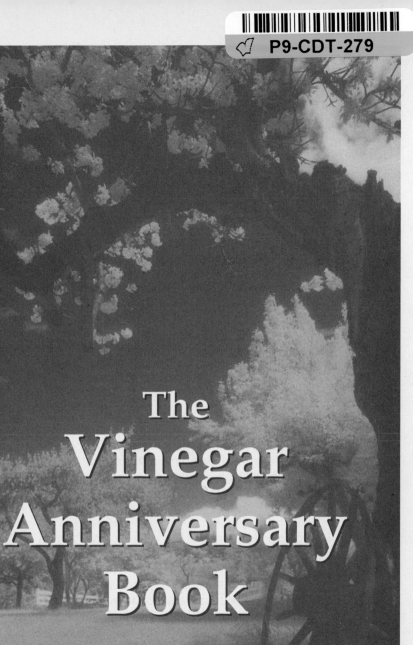

The Vinegar Anniversary Book

By Emily Thacker

A Very Special
Letter To My Readers

Dear Reader,

Thank you for your interest in this book and the others in the series. Your response to my previous books has been phenomenal. THE VINEGAR BOOK has more than 4,000,000 copies in print, in many languages and in more than a dozen countries. Your many letters are a continuing encouragement, filled with kind words and examples of how you, too, use vinegar and other natural home remedies.

Over many years and many books, we have shared a multitude of old-time ways. Together, we have explored legends, folklore and home remedies as well as scientific and medical findings. We have, especially, shared ways to use apple cider vinegar as part of better health and easier, safer cleaning. And, I cannot begin to tell you how many kind readers have written to me, asking for more vinegar information.

In reading my mail, it seems as if many of you feel apple cider vinegar is practically an instant remedy for all the ills of human kind. Some believe it is a liquid cure-all that can extend life, promote good health and provide needed vitamins, amino acids and trace elements. Faith in the power of apple cider vinegar dates back to about the time of the discovery of the apple. And, some of the claims made for it do seem to be a bit extravagant.

Do I feel apple cider vinegar is a remedy for all the ills of this world? Well, probably not.

Vinegar does contain a multitude of essential trace elements. Scientists have not yet decided on the exact amounts our bodies need of many of these valuable nutrients. The importance of these trace elements continues to be uncovered by medical scientists. Still, evidence continues to mount that pure, natural foods are our best source for both minerals and vitamins.

Newest findings show the number of elements and compounds in a good apple cider vinegar makes the ingredient list of most multivitamins look paltry by comparison. And, with the help of your contributions we have documented a multitude of vinegar based cleaning solutions. Vinegar is kind to the planet; this makes it unique among both food supplements and cleaning products.

Your letters have shown me your deep and continuing interest in the healthy benefits of vinegar. In reading them I have discovered much wisdom and found that I have left some questions about vinegar unanswered. This book brings together, in one comprehensive volume, the information presented in my four earlier vinegar books and combines it with the newest findings in vinegar research. So, whether you:

- Take a daily vinegar tonic
- Use vinegar in cooking
- Appreciate vinegar's value as a cleaning agent
- Apply vinegar as a disinfectant
- Count on vinegar to keep you healthy
- Use vinegar as an external pain reliever

… or simply enjoy vinegar's taste and its ties with the past … this book is dedicated to you, dear reader.

Wishing you all the best,

Emily

3

Table of Contents

What, Exactly, Is Vinegar?

S oon after the first person played a flute in Egypt—
About the time sheep were domesticated in the Near East—
As Europeans were learning to catch fish in nets of hair—
Before dogs were domesticated in the British Isles—

— Mankind discovered that a very useful, sour liquid formed
when a mildly alcoholic beverage was allowed to set out,
exposed to air. Vinegar came into being! And for more than
10,000 years it has been one of the most useful and widely
distributed liquids on the planet. Vinegar is, literally, soured
wine. When a sweet liquid, such as apple or grape juice, is
sealed up and allowed to ferment (away from air) the sugar in
it is changed into alcohol. If this liquid is permitted to ferment
for a second time (this time in the presence of air) the alcohol
is transformed into acetic acid. While the very first vinegar
came from the natural souring of fermented wine, it soon
became such a prized product that mankind learned how to
make it intentionally. Since then it has been used as a flavor
enhancing condiment, a preservative and as a cleaning agent
for people, pets and objects around the home.

WHAT IS VINEGAR?

Vinegar, with all its life-enhancing qualities, has been
used and appreciated since the most ancient of times.
Technically, vinegar is formed by the oxidation-fermentation
of ethanol, resulting in a brew which contains from 4% to
8% acetic acid. The ethanol (ethyl alcohol) is changed into
acetic acid (vinegar) through the growth of an acetobacter, a
living substance that eats (oxidizes) the alcohol and produces
(excretes) acetic acid. A good, naturally produced vinegar
contains far more than simply acetic acid. The acetobacter's

5

actions pack the fluid with newly created enzymes, while retaining particles of the food used to make the vinegar. The final result, that wonderful thing we call vinegar, has some of the goodness of the original food, enhanced with traces of a wonderful variety of vitamins, minerals and enzymes.

Enzymes have the ability to cause chemical reactions to take place without becoming directly involved in the process themselves. Vinegar's enzymes are made by living bacteria (acetobacter) and because they are catalysts for important biological chemical reactions, they are critical to life. As foods are turned into vinegar, they often pick up particles of other substances along the way. For example, naturally processed vinegar is often stored for several years in wooden casks. This contributes to its virtues, as can be seen by the way the flavor of the vinegar is changed by the type of wood used to make the barrels.

It was not until 1878, nearly 10,000 years after intentional vinegar making began, that a microbiologist named Hansen correctly explained the chemical process that creates vinegar. He accurately described the three species of vinegar bacilli, which are the tiny creatures that gobble up alcohol and excrete acid. The process where alcohols are changed to acids is called fermentation.

Many believe the fermentation process gives food a special ability to heal. It is also thought to sharply increase nutritional values. While the primary reason for fermenting foodstuffs was, originally, to keep them from rotting, the result can taste better than the original – just ask anyone who loves pickles.

Vinegar contains dilute acetic acid. It also has the basic nature and essential nutrients of the original food from which it was made. For example, apple cider vinegar has pectin, beta carotene and potassium from the apples that were its origin. In addition, it contains generous portions of health promoting enzymes and amino acids. These complex protein building blocks are formed during the fermentation process.

Claims for the curative and restorative powers of apple cider vinegar are legendary. Some believe this fabulous liquid is capable of solving the most vexing and tiresome of human afflictions. It has been said to lengthen life and improve hearing, vision and mental powers. Devotees claim it will help heartburn, clear up throat irritations, stop hiccups, relieve coughs, deal with diarrhea and ease asthma.

WHAT IS IN VINEGAR?

Vinegar has been credited with having a surprising number of health-promoting qualities. Many believe this is because of its unique combination of ingredients. For example, when apple cider vinegar is exposed to heat and air, it gives off some hints of its remarkable character. Take a healthy sniff and what you inhale is the 'volatile' part of vinegar, the portion that will evaporate easily. Scientists recently analyzed this small part of what vinegar is using gas chromatography-mass spectrometry. Amazingly, they were able to identify more than 90 compounds. Vinegar has:

7   Hydrocarbons
18 Alcohols
33 Carbonyls (4 aldehydes and 29 ketones)
4   Acids
8   Esters (plus 11 lactone esters)
7   Bases
3   Furans
13 Phenols

Distilled vinegar, usually considered to be the least nutritious of all vinegars, is a surprising storehouse of goodness. It has no fat, less than 30 calories and only 2 milligrams of sodium in an entire cup! Plus, it has a bit of protein, fiber and carbohydrate, plus calcium, phosphorus, iron, potassium, vitamins A and D, folacin, zinc, thiamin (vitamin B-1), riboflavin (vitamin B-2), niacin, magnesium and ascorbic acid (vitamin C).

The fine particles in cloudy vinegar contain tiny fragments of the original food from which it was made, so each variety has a unique nutritional content. In vinegars that have been filtered, these particles are usually not visible. Organic vinegar may look a bit cloudy and have a layer of sediment in the bottom of the bottle. This is a sign the product has not had precious nutrients filtered or precipitated out.

Apples in apple cider vinegar bring amino acids such as tryptophan, threonine, isoleucine, leucine, lysine, methionine, cystine, phenylalanine, tyrosine, valine, arginine, histidine, alanine, aspartic acid, glutamic acid, glycine, proline and serine. And they bring vitamins such as A, B-6, folate, asorbic acid, thiamin, riboflavin, niacin and pantothenic acid. Plus, apples have minerals such as calcium, iron, magnesium, phosphorus, potassium, zinc, copper and manganese. So, while vinegar contains everything found in acetic acid, it also contains much more.

The exact composition of a particular vinegar depends on what plant product it was made from. Even apple cider vinegar varies with the kind and condition of the apples in it. Partly because of this, medical scientists do not always know exactly how or why it promotes healing. They do know that all vinegar is both antiseptic and antibiotic.

HOW VINEGAR IS MADE

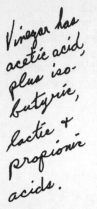

Vinegar has acetic acid, plus iso-butyric, lactic + propionic acids.

The history of vinegar making is as old as that of mankind. The first vinegar probably began as wine that was exposed to air. Wild yeasts fermented it into a wonderful, life-enhancing liquid! For centuries vinegar was thought to be a magically created potion. Those who knew how to oversee and control the making of the wondrous brew guarded the secret carefully, then handed the process down to their children – because, all vinegar is not created equal. Its aroma and flavor are influenced by the way it is made and aged.

Vinegar is a complex substance, brimming with subtle flavors and aromas and packed with an assortment of nutrients, enzymes and trace elements. The best vinegar is a combination of sweet mellowness from wooden storage barrels and the sharp, sour zing of acetic acid. The flavor, aroma and healthfulness of vinegar are supplied by the food from which it is made, and from the container used for aging it. Vinegar can be made from any plant that contains enough sugar to ferment into the alcohol needed to make acetic acid. That food should have a pleasant flavor and aroma, as these beginning qualities will carry over into the finished product and contribute to the final taste and flavor of the vinegar. Vinegar production begins when a sugary liquid is changed into an alcoholic one by yeast. Then, this brew is changed into an acetic acid containing solution. The microorganisms that cause the alcohol to change to acetic acid are those of the Acetobacter group.

VINEGAR MAKING

To make good apple cider vinegar begin with freshly washed whole apples, chopped or coarsely ground. (Apple cider vinegar can also be made from just cores and peelings.) Include both tart and sweet apples for full flavor and aroma. A few crab apples tossed in will add a bit of zip. Allow the chopped apples to set briefly, so the cut apples begin to react with the air and form the tannins which give it rich color and deep flavor. Press the juice from the apples, let it ferment into hard cider, then ferment again into vinegar. Adding a dab of mother-of-vinegar (mother) to the cider will hurry the process along.

The particular bacteria which produces vinegar is called acetobacter. This gooey glob, called mother, floats on the surface. These good bacteria feed on oxygen and reproduce rapidly in substances that meet their nutritional needs. Acetobacter tends to continuously change into new forms, so those who want to produce a standardized product use a starter, just as a yeast starter is used in making bread.

Wine vinegar, like wine, can begin with either red or white grapes. Red wine vinegar is flavorful and intense, whereas white is apt to be a bit more astringent. Before processing and the standardization of its acid content wine vinegar has a higher natural concentration of acetic acid than apple cider vinegar. This is because grapes have a higher sugar content than apples.

Some people use cores, peelings and windfalls.

Balsamic vinegar is specially aged Italian wine vinegar. It is very dark, strongly aromatic and sweet. This is considered to be the very best, most concentrated vinegar.

Sherry vinegar is a brownish amber color and has the woodsy, nutty taste and fragrance of Spanish sherry. It is not as sweet-tasting as apple cider vinegar.

Champagne vinegar is made from grapes picked before they are fully ripe. This vinegar is mild and delicate, which makes it a good choice as a base for flower-scented vinegars.

Malt vinegar begins with barley, which is soaked in water, allowed to germinate and is then fermented into this dark English favorite. It is a robust, full-flavored vinegar and an essential ingredient of Worcestershire sauce.

Rice vinegar, at its best, most nutritious, is made from whole rice. Cost conscious producers sometimes make lower grades from the lees left after the manufacture of rice wine. Rice vinegar is one of the mildest kinds and can be clear, red or dark brown in color. It is an integral part of both oriental cooking and Traditional Chinese Medicine (TCM).

Life is a natural process. Your vinegar should be natural, too.

Organic vinegar indicates a product that is produced without chemical additives, from food which has been grown without the use of pesticides. And, good organic vinegar should contain obvious remnants of the healthful food from which it was made. It should be a product that has not had its goodness filtered out, and not been over heated or over processed. Because organic vinegar can sometimes contain beneficial sediment at the bottom the bottle, it may not be as 'pretty' as pasteurized, super-filtered varieties.

A Word About Heat . . .
When using organic products that have not been pasteurized to make specialty vinegars, do not use heat, as it can harm nutrients. Heat can also deplete aromatics.

Acetic is not the only acid formed during vinegar production. Some newly formed acids react with residual traces of alcohol and form esters. Esters are important to creating the unique, individual aroma of various vinegars. Some facts about making, storing and using vinegar follow:

VINEGAR AND FIBER

Vinegar – particularly fortified vinegar – contains a treasure trove of complex carbohydrates, as well as a good dose of that mysterious stuff called "dietary fiber." Both complex carbohydrates and dietary fiber have been recommended by the U.S. Surgeon General to help build resistance to cancer.

Yes, there are different kinds of fibers. Some are water soluble and some are not. A water soluble fiber soaks up water (adding bulk) but also has the power to interact with the body. Insoluble fibers soak up water (adding bulk) but do not interact with the body in the same complex way soluble fibers do.

Wheat bran is only 56% digestible.

When vinegar is made from fresh, natural apples it contains a healthy dose of pectin. Pectin is a soluble fiber. It dissolves in water, making it very available for the body to use. In addition to soaking up water, it slows down the absorption of food and liquid in the intestines. Therefore, it stays in the body longer than an insoluble fiber.

An insoluble fiber, such as wheat bran, rushes through the system. Particularly, it rushes through the intestines. This gives it laxative properties. Wheat bran may also produce large amounts of gas. As pectin (apple cider vinegar fiber) works its slow, gentle way through the digestive system it binds to cholesterol. Then pectin pulls the cholesterol that is bound to it out of the body. Less cholesterol in the body makes for a reduced risk of cardiovascular problems, such as heart attacks and strokes.

Natural, organic vinegars are not the same as commercially processed and pasteurized products. In its most natural state vinegar is alive with living organisms. These naturally occurring creatures, as well as some enzymes and vitamins are destroyed when vinegar is processed in a high heat process, such as pasteurization. Descriptions of a couple of these little inhabitants of the vinegar barrel follow:

Vinegar eels are frequently found in vinegar. This species of nematode worm is a natural part of many vinegars. These curious creatures can be seen near the surface of vinegar that has been exposed to air. They resemble tiny threadworms and are considered a harmless part of vinegar.

Vinegar flies (of the genus Drosophila) lay eggs that hatch out into larvae that live comfortably in vinegar. They thrive on this acid brew, but are not a particularly appetizing addition to vinegar!

For thousands of years apple cider vinegar has been made in much the same way. First, cider is made from a specially selected assortment of whole, fresh apples: they are washed, chopped, and pressed.

When the sweet apple juice has been collected, it is allowed to age, sealed tightly away from the air. Natural sugars are fermented to produce alcohol. This "hard" cider is then allowed to ferment once again, while left open to the air. This time, the alcohol changes to acid.

Originally, the commercial production of vinegar was a by-product of the wine producer and the brewer. Vinegar brewing, as a separate industry, dates from about the 17th century. First established in France, it quickly spread to other regions.

Vinegar can be made from any liquid containing sugar, if there is enough sugar. Apple juice is one of the oldest fluids used to make vinegar, but grape and date palm use goes back thousands of years. Other popular vinegar sources are: molasses, sorghum, berries, melons, coconuts, honey, maple syrup, potatoes, beets, grains, bananas, and even whey.

Wine vinegar has many of the same nutritional benefits as apple cider vinegar. After all, it begins with naturally ripe, vitamin and mineral packed fruit. Wine vinegar will vary in color, depending on whether it was made from red or white wine. Vinegar's flavor, strength and nutritional makeup depend on what it is made from.

Alegar
One of the old-time vinegars made from a grain base is called alegar. Technically, it is a kind of malt vinegar. Malt is barley (or other grain) which is steeped in water until it germinates, then dried in a kiln for use in brewing. This malt is fermented into an alcoholic beverage called ale. Ale has less hops than beer, so it is both sweeter and lighter

in color.

The color of alegar varies from pale gold to rich brown. The intensity of the color depends on how the grain was roasted and dried. Medicated herbal ales have been used for hundreds of years in Europe.

MOTHER OF VINEGAR

Mother (or mother-of-vinegar) is the term used to describe the mass of sticky scum that forms on top of cider (or other juice) when alcohol turns into vinegar. As the fermentation progresses, mother forms a gummy, stringy, floating lump. Mother is formed by the beneficial bacteria that create vinegar.

The particular kind of bacteria that produces vinegar is called acetobacter. This gooey glob, called mother, floats on the surface. These good bacteria feed on oxygen and reproduce rapidly in substances that meet their nutritional needs. Acetobacter tends to continuously change into new forms, so those who want to produce a standardized product use a starter, just as a yeast starter is used in making bread. Acetic is not the only acid formed during vinegar production. Some newly formed acids react with residual traces of alcohol and form esters. Esters are important to creating the unique, individual aroma of various vinegars.

Fortunately the vinegaroon — a large scorpion — does not live in vinegar.

Sometimes mother from a previous batch of vinegar is introduced into another liquid that is in the process of becoming vinegar. This use, as a starter for new vinegars, is why the gooey scum on the top of vinegar is called mother-of-vinegar. Sometimes, as mother begins to form, it is disturbed and sinks to the bottom of the container. If it falls into the vinegar it will die, because its oxygen supply is cut off. This dead, slithery blob is called a zoogloea and is worthless.

Mother sinks for two reasons. First, if the vinegar making container is jolted, the film can get wet. This makes it too heavy to float. Second, if too many tiny vinegar eels develop in the liquid, their weight, as they cling to the edges of the developing mother, will weight it down.

Over the ages, traditional vinegar makers developed a deep reverence for the rubbery mass of goo we call mother-of-vinegar. Often, some was saved from a batch of vinegar. Then, it was

12

transferred carefully to new batches of souring wine to work its magic. Over time, this cultivated mother developed special flavoring abilities. It is still handed down, from generation to generation and guarded as a secret ingredient in special vinegars. Tiny bits of the old mother are lifted out of one batch of vinegar and put into new batches.

Mother-of-vinegar may also form on stored vinegar supplies. This slime is not particularly appealing, but its presence does not mean the vinegar is spoiled. Skim it off and use the vinegar.

MAKE YOUR OWN VINEGAR

There are as many ways to make vinegar as there are apples, kinds of fruit, and people. If you have never tackled the operation, you may want to begin with the first apple cider vinegar recipe below. Then, try some of the other ways to make vinegar.

Vinegar making requires two separate, distinct fermentations. The first, called alcoholic (or vinous) changes natural sugars to alcohol. The second, called acid (or acetic) changes alcohol to acetic acid. It is important that the first fermenting be completely finished before the second is begun.

You can hurry the first fermentation along by adding a little yeast to the cider, and by keeping it warm. At around 80° the liquids will convert very fast. To speed up the second fermentation, add a little mother-of-vinegar to the mix. And, the more air the mixture gets during this second part of the process, the faster it will convert to vinegar.

Acetous fermentation is how alcoholic liquids, like beer or wine, yield acetic acid.

Caution: Mother-of-vinegar (it starts the second fermentation) must not get into the liquid until practically all the sugar has been converted to alcohol.

The vinegar bacterium is present wherever there is air. This is why any wine which is spilled at a winery must be mopped up at once. Bacteria could get started in the wine and sour it all! If a winery makes both wine and vinegar, separate rooms are used for each. And, barrels from vinegar making are never used for storing wine.

Apple Cider Vinegar

Begin by making a good, tart cider. Combine sweet apples for aroma, tart ones for body, and a few crab apples for luck. The more sweet apples you use, the stronger the vinegar will be. This is because

13

the high sugar content of sweet apples produces more alcohol to change into acid. The more tart apples in the mix, the sharper the flavor will be.

Chop the apples and when they turn golden brown, crush them in a cider press. Collect the cider in a glass jug. Never use store-bought apple juice to make vinegar. It may not ferment properly!

Next, cap the cider jug with a small balloon. It will expand as carbon dioxide is released, while keeping air away from the mix. When the sugar is all changed to alcohol, it becomes hard cider. This takes 1 to 6 weeks, depending on the temperature and the sugar content of the apples used to make the cider. It is not necessary to add yeast, as wild yeasts are always on apples' surfaces and in the air. If a gray foam forms on the top of the cider, it is excess yeast, and is harmless. Just skim it off.

Finally, pour the hard cider into a wide crock, so there is a larger surface area than in a jug. Put a cloth over the top to let in air, while keeping out dust and bugs. Vinegar will be created in a few months.

Wild spores floating in the air will start the fermenting process, but adding mother-of-vinegar to the cider will hurry the conversion along. Simply smear a slice of toast with mother and lay it gently on the surface of the cider. Vinegar making works best if the ingredients are kept at around 80°. If the temperature gets very much higher, the bacteria needed for fermenting is killed. If the temperature gets much cooler than 80°, the spores will become dormant.

Other Old Apple Cider Vinegar Recipes

Put cut up apples in a stone crock and cover them with warm water. Tie a cheesecloth over the top and set in a warm place for 4-6 months. Then strain off the vinegar. For faster action, add a lump of raw bread dough to the crock.

Place apple and peach peelings and a handful of grape skins in a wide mouth jar and cover these fruit leavings with cold water. Set in a warm place and add a couple of fresh apple cores every few days. When a scum forms on top, stop adding fresh fruit and let it thicken. When the vinegar is good and strong, strain it through a cheesecloth. Speed up the process by adding brown sugar, molasses or yeast.

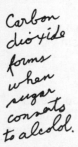
Carbon dioxide forms when sugar consorts to alcohol.

Other Vinegars

Let a bottle of wine stand, open to the air, in the summer sun. In about 2 weeks it will turn into a nice vinegar. Make winter vinegar by letting wine stand open to the air for about a month. Put 2 pounds of golden raisins in a gallon of water and set it in a warm place. In 2 months it will become white wine vinegar. Just strain the vinegar off and bottle it. Make some more vinegar by adding another 1/2 pound of raisins to the dredges and going through the process again.

Make a deeply colored honey vinegar by pouring 1 gallon boiling water over 5 pounds of strained honey. Stir until all of the honey is melted. Then dissolve 1 cake (or package) of yeast in 1 tablespoon of warm water. Spread the yeast on a dry corn cob (or a slice of toast) and float it on the top of the honey-water. Cover the container with a cloth and let it set for 16 days. Take out the corn cob, skim off the scum and strain the liquid. Now let it stand for a month or so, until it turns into vinegar.

Dark, strong flavored honeys will ferment much faster than light, mild ones. Add a cup or two of fruit juice or molasses to the honey to speed up the change to vinegar. Because the sugar content of honey varies a lot, you may want to check and see if your water-to honey ratio is correct. Do this by dropping an egg into the mixture. It should float in the liquid, with only a small spot showing above the surface. If the egg sinks, add more honey. If the egg floats too high, add more water. This method should assure you that the specific gravity of the mix is about 1.05, the best for making good honey vinegar.

For an extra special, clover-flavored, vinegar add a quart of freshly washed clover blossoms to the honey and water mix. Dandelions add a unique taste to honey vinegar. Just add 3 cups of blossoms to the honey and water. Be sure to strain it before using!

A Baume hydro-meter will read between 7 and 8.

Raspberry vinegar can be prepared by pouring 2 quarts of water over 1 quart of freshly washed red or black raspberries. Cover lightly and let stand overnight. Strain off the liquid and discard the berries. Now prepare 1 more quart of fresh raspberries and pour the same liquid over them. Let this set overnight. Do this for a total of 5 times. Then add 1 pound of sugar to the liquid and stir until it is dissolved. Set the mixture aside, uncovered, for a couple of months. Strain before using.

HOW STRONG IS YOUR HOMEMADE VINEGAR?

Commercial vinegar's acid content is standardized, but homemade vinegars can vary. What follows is one way to determine the percent of acid in a batch of vinegar. You will need 1/2 cup water

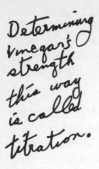
Determining vinegar's strength this way is called titration.

and 2 teaspoons baking soda, mixed together, plus, 1/4 cup of the water in which a head of red cabbage was cooked.

- Put 1/2 cup water into each of 2 clear glasses.
- Add 1/8 cup cabbage water to each glass.
- Use a glass dropper to put 7 drops of commercial vinegar into one glass of the cabbage flavored water.
- Rinse the dropper.
- Put 20 drops of the soda water into the same glass and stir well (stir with a plastic spoon, not metal). The water will turn blue.
- Now mix 7 drops of your vinegar into the second glass of the cabbage flavored water.
- Rinse the dropper.
- Add baking soda water to your vinegar and cabbage water, 1 drop at a time. Stir after each drop. Count the drops.
- When the color of your vinegar water turns the same shade of blue as the commercial vinegar water, the acid content of the two glasses will match.

Wash fruit for vinegar making.

To find the percent of acid in your vinegar, divide the number of drops of soda water you added to it by four. For example, if you added 20 drops of soda water to your vinegar, divide by four and find that the acid content is 5%. (The same as most commercial vinegars.) The more soda water it takes to make your vinegar match the color of the commercial vinegar control, the stronger your vinegar is.

HOW NOT TO MAKE VINEGAR

Vinegar producers of the 1800's found they could make acetic acid from wood chips, or even from the residues discarded during paper making. These companies added flavorings and color and called the result apple cider vinegar. This cheap imitation was, of course, deficient in taste and aroma and did not contain the vast array of natural enzymes and nutrients of the original. today's labeling laws prevent this kind of product adulteration - if the bottle says apple cider vinegar - it contains vinegar that began life as apples.

Got Vinegar?
History's Uses

*O*ur word 'vinegar' comes from the French 'vinaigre,' VIN meaning wine and IGRE meaning sour. And that is just what it is: wine that has gone sour. According to the Associated Press, vinegar is "an organic molecule that may have played a role in the formation of life." Scientists agree that vinegar had an important role in the creation of life. They tell us it was part of the primordial soup that provided a chemical start for life because when vinegar is combined with ammonia, it makes up the simplest biologically important building block of life.

This is why scientists were excited when astronomers at the University of Illinois found vinegar in the cloud of gas and dust called Sagittarius B2 North. *USA Today* put it this way, by reporting that vinegar had been "found in a cloud of dust and gas 25,000 light years from earth." *Science Digest* tells us vinegar is a "building block for the body" and the *New York Herald Tribune* says it is "used by the body to burn fat."

Many people believe that taking a bit of vinegar each day is vitally important for a healthy, vital body. For example, one television evangelist claims that taking a daily tonic that includes vinegar helped him gain the strength to leg press more than a 1,000 pounds!

A VINEGAR'S BEGINNINGS

Vinegars get most of their unique taste from acetic acid, but they contain much more. When foods go through the double fermentation process that produces vinegar the result is a liquid laced with trace amounts of newly created alcohols, phenols and enzymes. And yet, according to the World Health Organization, they retain tiny particles of the original food. This can include their natural store of vitamins and minerals.

All vinegar begins as pure wholesome food. It is made from apples, grapes, rice, barley, bananas, or any one of dozens of other healthy foods. Vinegar can be made of any food with enough sugar content to ferment into the alcohol needed to create it. Some of the many foods which are used to make vinegar include: apples, apricots, bananas, barley, beets, blackberries, cane, coconut, corn, cranberries, dates, grapes, guava, honey, mangoes, maple syrup, molasses, oats, oranges, papaya, passion fruit, peaches, pears, persimmons, pineapples, plums, raspberries, rice, strawberries, sweet potatoes, watermelons, whey or white potatoes.

If you begin with:	You get this vinegar:
Apples	Apple Cider
Grapes	Wine or Champagne
Rice	Rice
Barley	Malt
Bananas	Banana

We associate vinegar made with particular foods with certain countries. For example:

Apples	United States
Dates	Ancient Babylonia
Bananas	Nicaragua
Malt	England
Cane	Philippines
Potatoes	Germany
Rice	China (and Japan)
Coconut	Indonesia

Vinegar is made from many substances. For industrial uses, acetic acid that has been manufactured from wood products is diluted to make a kind of vinegar. At one time this colorless product was colored with caramel and sold as table grade vinegar, although its food value and aroma were inferior to food based vinegar. Today, this adulterated vinegar is rarely sold as a food.

WHERE DID VINEGAR COME FROM?

3,000 years before barley is grown to make beer, 4,000 years before all of Mesopotamia is engulfed in a disastrous flood, 5,000 years before wheeled vehicles appear in Sumeria or the Egyptians learn to plow, an enterprising householder prepares some fresh, naturally sweetened juice and seals it tightly in a stone jar. In a short time it ferments into the mildly intoxicating brew we call wine.

A very special day soon follows. The wine is left open to the air. A second fermentation takes place. Vinegar is created! Imagine the surprise of the poor soul who took the first sip of this new brew. All the alcohol in the wine had turned into a sharp tasting acid! Had a partially filled wine cask been unknowingly set aside and left uncared for? Had a servant carelessly left the wine uncorked? Or could it possibly be ... did someone suspect the possibilities?

Although we do not know exactly how it happened, vinegar had been discovered and the result was historic! It was found to be an almost universal preservative and cure-all. Vegetables could be kept indefinitely in this wonderful liquid and fish remained edible long after they should have rotted. Festering wounds began to heal when soaked in this remarkable fluid. It only followed that mankind would confer an exalted status to this amazing concoction. After all, it changed the way mankind ate and fought germs for all time!

It has been at least 10,000 years since the natural souring of wine created the first vinegar.

Vinegar accomplishes all this because it inhibits the growth of microorganisms that cause food to spoil and infection to spread. Some of this is due to its acid, which prevents microbial growth. The newly formed chemicals in vinegar improve flavor, too. Vinegar also has nonacid preserving qualities, as do salt, sugar and spices, which are sometimes added to vinegar to boost its ability to preserve.

VINEGAR'S EARLIEST MEDICAL USES

This naturally occurring germ killer was one of the very first medicines. The Babylonians, back in 5,000 B.C., fermented the fruits of the date palm. Their vinegar, therefore, was called date vinegar and was credited with having

19

superior healing properties.

An early Assyrian medical text described the treatment for ear pain as being the application of vinegar. In 400BC, Hippocrates (considered the Father of Medicine) used vinegar to treat his patients.

Vinegar was used as a healing dressing on wounds and infectious sores in Bible Times. Thieves Vinegar got its name during the time of the Great Plague of Europe. Some enterprising thieves are said to have used vinegar to protect them from contamination while they robbed the homes of plague victims. Vinegar is credited with saving the lives of thousands of soldiers during the U.S. Civil War, where it was routinely used as a disinfectant on wounds.

VINEGAR AND THE SKIN

Historically, infections on the face, around the eyes and in the ears have been treated with a solution of vinegar and water. It works because vinegar is antiseptic (it kills germs on contact) and antibiotic (it contains bacteria which is unfriendly to infectious microorganisms).

Once the ancient world recognized vinegar's value for healing and health, the intentional production of this amazing elixir began. Because vinegar could do so many miraculous things it is not surprising that the souring of apple cider into vinegar was often an elaborate process, with overtones of magic.

Vinegar making was, for thousands of years, more an art form than a science. The physical steps for making vinegar were often augmented with incantations and seemingly superfluous steps.

We now know the complicated recipes of the medieval alchemists were not needed. These early recipes owed their success to the accidental infection of their brews with organisms needed for fermentation. It was exposure to air that brought vinegar into being!

VINEGAR'S HISTORIC DEVELOPMENT

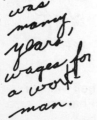

As vinegar's virtues became known, its production spread throughout the world. Vinegar's use can be chronicled down through the ages in many different times and cultures. It has been used for everyday cleaning and for specific medical ailments for at least 10,000 years. And sometimes, vinegar can be said to have actually changed the course of history. Some of the more intriguing historic vinegar uses, as well as some vinegar hints for today, follow.

Hannibal & Vinegar

Was vinegar the worlds first bulldozer? Without vinegar, Hannibal's march over the Alps to Rome may not have been possible! The chronicles of this historic march describe the essential role vinegar played in the task of getting Hannibal's elephants over the perilous mountain trails.

Frequently, the torturous passage across the Alps was too narrow for the huge elephants. Hannibal's solution was for his soldiers to cut tree limbs and stack them around the boulders that blocked their way. Then the limbs were set afire. When the rocks were good and hot, vinegar was poured onto them. This turned the stones soft and crumbly. The soldiers could then chip the rocks away, making a passage for both the troops and elephants that helped make Hannibal famous.

The Most Expensive Meal Ever

The world's most costly meal may have begun with a glass of vinegar. When asked to think of the most expensive beverage, vinegar may not come immediately to mind. Yet it may take the prize for most expensive drink in history! Cleopatra, queen of Egypt, made culinary history when she made a wager that she could consume, at a single meal, the value of a million sisterces. To many, it seemed an impossible task. After all, how could anyone eat so much?

Cleopatra was able to consume a meal worth so very much by dropping a million sisterces worth of pearls into a glass of vinegar. Then she set it aside while banquet preparations were made. When the time came to fulfill her wager, she simply drank the dissolved pearls!

Other Historic Vinegar Moments

You may know that vinegar is mentioned several times in the Bible. (in both the Old Testament and in the New Testament.) But did you know there was a Vinegar Bible?

One famous version of the Bible is called the Vinegar Bible. In 1717 the Clarendon Press in Oxford, England printed and released a new edition of the scriptures. A mistake was soon discovered. In the top-of-the-page running headline of the 22nd chapter of the book of Luke, the word "vineyard" had been misprinted. Instead of "vineyard" the printer typeset the word as "vinegar." The edition was quickly dubbed the "Vinegar Bible." And this is the name by which Clarendon's

1717 edition is known today.

Even poets have commented on vinegar. Lord Byron (1788-1824) called vinegar "A sad, sour, sober beverage..."

KINDS OF VINEGAR

Distilled, or white vinegar is usually used for cleaning. Because white vinegar is a colorless liquid it is less likely to discolor articles being cleaned. Generally, white vinegar is made from wood or grain and has a consistent 5% acetic acid content.

White vinegar is often used for pickling, salad dressings, marinating and for preparing foods when the distinctive flavor of other vinegars is not wanted. It is a reliable, consistent, inexpensive and widely available product. For most cooking, when special flavor is wanted, or for personal use, other kinds of vinegar are usually used. Apple cider is widely available, inexpensive, has a long history of health uses and has a fresh, distinctive flavor.

Herbal and balsamic vinegars are more expensive and harder to find. Balsamic vinegar is aged in wood, often for several years. It is considered one of the finest flavorings available for many foods. Herbal vinegars can usually be found in health food stores. Or, they can be prepared from white, apple cider or wine vinegar. Vinegars made by old, slower processes are known for their fine aromas and have more subtle flavors than ones made by newer, faster processes. Aromatic vinegars have spices and herbs added to them. They produce a fragrant liquid that is used in the kitchen and in personal care products such as after shave lotions and skin fresheners.

Descriptions of the most popular vinegars, plus when and how to use them follow:

White (distilled) vinegar is made from any product leftovers that are cheap and plentiful. It does not have exactly the same components and tantalizing aroma of more expensive specialty vinegars, but can be used for pickling. It is the best choice for preserving the whiteness of foods such as cauliflower and white onions. And, since it has little flavor of its own, it is sometimes used in making vinegars flavored with delicate herbs. This most inexpensive of vinegars is the best choice for cleaning.

Apple cider vinegar is the most typically American vinegar. This apple-based product is a good, healthy general purpose product. It is a great choice for most pickling, cooking and skin care. In taste it is similar to, but more tart than, rice vinegar.

Balsamic vinegar has been produced for the past 800 years in the Modena region of Italy. It is considered the greatest of all vinegars, and thought by many to have medicinal properties. In Italy, aceto balsamico is known as "the healthful vinegar." Balsamic vinegar is a wine vinegar that is aged until its vinegary tartness is overlaid with sweetness and flavor it absorbs from a succession of wooden storage barrels.

The best balsamic vinegars are as expensive and aged as long as good wine. They slowly evaporate and become concentrated, not merely with a higher acidic content, but with richer, more intense flavors. This vinegar begins with grapes that have an extremely high sugar content, making it sweet, rich, thick and brown-colored. The grapes are cooked before processing to concentrate their juice. Then the vinegar is aged in a succession of wooden barrels. The kind of wood influences the ultimate flavor. Many balsamic vinegars are aged 50 years or more. It is dark brown and has more body than other types.

JAPANESE RICE VINEGAR AND HEALTH

Taking vinegar and honey as a life enhancing tonic is more than merely an American custom. In Japan it is an old favorite, too. Japan's most famous vinegar is made from rice. The bulk of Japanese commercial vinegar is made from wine leftovers. The sediment left from the production of the rice wine called sake is used to make industrial vinegar. These dregs, called lees produce a vinegar which is similar in nutrient value to our white vinegar.

The rice vinegar that is used for cooking and healing remedies is made directly from brown rice. Belief in the healing nature of this deeply colored rice vinegar has come down through thousands of years of Japanese culture.

Some ways of using vinegar that have endured for centuries - and some of Japan's newest research into the healing power of rice vinegar follow:

According to the Japan Food Research Laboratories, vinegar made directly from brown rice has five times the amount of amino acids as the commercial product made from lees. Perhaps the healthful benefits of rice vinegar are because of the

Vinegar fights free radicals that cause aging.

23

20 amino acids it contains. Or maybe it is the sixteen organic acids that can be found in it.

The bottom of the bottle of even the best rice vinegar will have a fine rice sediment. When these grounds are disturbed they give the vinegar a muddy appearance. This dark residue is considered to be the mark of a high quality rice vinegar.

Recent research by Dr. Yoshio Takino, of Shizuka University in Japan, proved vinegar helps to maintain good health and slow down aging by helping to prevent the formation of two fatty peroxides. This is important to good health and long life in two important ways. One is associated with damaging free radicals; the other with the cholesterol formations that build up on blood vessel walls.

In Japan, vinegar is used to produce one of that country's most potent folk remedies. Tamago-su, or egg vinegar is made by immersing a whole, raw egg in a cup of rice vinegar. The egg and vinegar are allowed to set, undisturbed, for seven days. During this time the vinegar dissolves the egg, shell and all. At the end of one week the only part of the egg which has not been dissolved is the transparent membrane, located just inside the shell. The Tamago-su maker splits open this membrane and dumps its contents into the glass of vinegar. This piece of the egg is discarded and what remains is thoroughly mixed.

A small amount of this very powerful egg vinegar is taken three times a day, stirred into a glass of hot water. It is believed it will assure a long, healthy life. Traditionally, Samurai warriors considered an egg vinegar tonic to be an important source of strength and power.

Vinegar is used as a bleaching agent on white vegetables. It also prevents enzymatic browning. When foods do not darken in air, they do not develop the off-taste associated with browning. Rice vinegar is also used in salad dressings, marinades, sauces, dips and spreads.

Without vinegar there would be no sushi.

Rice vinegar (like all vinegars) is a powerful antiseptic. It kills, on contact, dangerous bacteria such as salmonella and streptococcus.

The sushi industry is largely dependent on vinegar's ability to prevent germs from growing on the raw fish. It is sprinkled on the fish, included in dipping sauces and used as a preservative.

24

Vinegar acts as a tenderizer on meats and vegetables used in stir-fry dishes.

Japanese housewives add a little rice vinegar to summer rice to prevent it from spoiling.

Vinegar, added to fish dishes, helps to eliminate the traditional fishy odor. It also helps get rid of fish smells at clean up time.

WHAT KIND OF VINEGAR DO I USE?

Most cleaning chores call for white vinegar. Some food recipes call for white vinegar, others are better with apple cider (or even herbal or wine) vinegar. In most cases, the difference in vinegars is one of taste and aroma, not of effectiveness. In this volume, if a specific type of vinegar is best in a particular circumstance, the cleaning tip or recipe specifies the kind. If the kind of vinegar is not indicated, either white or apple cider vinegar may be used — the choice is yours!

Old-Time
Pain Relievers

5 0 years ago a daily apple cider vinegar and honey tonic was recommended to ease arthritis. During the past 30 years, 'wonder drugs' have replaced it and other folk remedies. Now, vinegar and many other old-time remedies are finding new followers, including many medical professionals. One reason for vinegar's renewed appeal is that almost everyone has experienced the negative side effects of today's powerful new drugs.

It is very possible this old remedy will, one day soon, be shown to desensitize the body to arthritis causing allergens as it strengthens the immune system. The immune system and arthritis have very strong ties because it mediates the body's power to heal and repair itself. A weak immune system does not aggressively repair cell damage. And, an undernourished immune system cannot tell the difference between invading germs and healthy body tissue. So, it attacks and destroys cartilage in joints. It also loses the ability to replace cartilage in joints as is worn away. But, it can be dangerous to take too much of some vitamins and minerals. For example, extra, unbalanced zinc in the body can deplete copper, another mineral long associated with arthritis. It can even bring about a suppression of the immune response. Most doctors agree the best way to add balanced vitamins and minerals to the immune system is with healthy foods. Apple cider vinegar has long been considered one way to do this.

VINEGAR AND ARTHRITIS

Arthritis sufferers spend $8 to $10 billion each year searching for relief – relief that, too often, does not come. Those who are feeling the pain of arthritis will try almost anything to be free of the disease. This often results in large sums of money being spent on supposed cures that do not improve health, relieve chronic pain or stop the progression of the disease.

The Select Committee on Aging's Subcommittee on Health and Long Term Care (House of Represen-tatives, 98th Congress) calls the marketing of supposed arthritis cures a $10 billion a year scandal. In reporting on this, the *Journal of the American Dietetic Association* notes that both medical and nutrition authorities agree on one important fact about arthritis care:

The only specific treatment for arthritis is "weight control ... and a nutrient-dense diet ...." This respected journal goes on to explain the conclusions nutritional scientists have drawn from studies of the eating habits of arthritis sufferers: Sometimes the patient's diet is found to be "... grossly deficient in some nutrients."

Perhaps this helps to explain the long-standing belief by many that apple cider vinegar can play an important part in relieving the pain and slowing the progression of arthritis. At the very least it is less likely to hurt the one taking it than some of the more outrageous chemicals which have been advertised as being able to ease the symptoms of arthritis. And, in addition, it is inexpensive!

The time-honored vinegar recipe for dealing with arthritis is 1 teaspoon honey and 1 teaspoon apple cider vinegar, mixed into a glass of water and taken morning and evening.

Apple cider vinegar is an old folk remedy for arthritis. The traditional way to take it is to mix a teaspoon of vinegar with a teaspoon of clover honey and stir them into a full glass of water. Drink this mixture two or three times a day. One reason this is thought to be of benefit to some people is that many of the elderly have marginal vitamin deficiencies. This is especially true for those taking medications for rheumatoid arthritis. Folic acid stores are especially likely to become depleted. Yet, arthritis' inflammation has been reduced when thiamin, B-6 and B-12 were added to standard medical treatments. Results could be seen in as little as one week!

Others believe the proper dose is to drink a glass of water, with 2 teaspoons vinegar in it, before each meal (3 times a day).

Another tonic that has often been recommended for those who suffer from arthritis' discomfort combines vinegar with celery, Epsom® salts, and citrus (for vitamin C). Combine in a saucepan:

1/2 grapefruit
1 orange
1 lemon
2 stalks celery
4 cups water
Cut the celery and fruit (including the peelings) into chunks. Simmer in water, uncovered, for 1 hour. Press the softened foods through a jelly bag and then stir in 1 tablespoon vinegar and 1 tablespoon Epsom® salts. Drink a full glass of water, morning and evening, to which 1/4 cup of this tonic has been added.

Witch hazel added to vinegar's effective- ness.

With any vinegar regimen, expect it to take about a month for relief to begin. For more immediate results, many doctors say a gentle rub down may help. One old-time liniment combines vinegar and oil with egg whites:

2 egg whites
1/2 cup turpentine
1/2 cup vinegar
1/4 cup olive oil
Mix all the ingredients together and use right away. Gently massage aching joints with this mixture, then wipe it off with a soft cloth. (Most medical authorities would recommend leaving the turpentine out of this remedy, as it can cause skin irritation.)

EASE PAIN & SUFFERING

Over the centuries vinegar became a commonplace remedy for many ills. Some examples of ancient recipes for health, well-being and sanitation follow:

Headaches will fade away if you follow this simple procedure: add a dash of apple cider vinegar to the water in a vaporizer and inhale the vapors for 5 minutes. Lay quietly and the headache should be relived in 20 minutes.

Hiccups will disappear if you sip, very slowly, a glass of warm water with 1 teaspoon of vinegar in it. This works even better if you sip from the far side of the glass!

An unsettled stomach will calm down if you sip quietly on a glass of very warm water, to which has been added 1 tablespoon honey and 1 tablespoon vinegar. This is also good for easing gas.

If a headache will not go away, try a paper bag hat. Soak the bottom of the open edges of a brown paper bag in apple cider vinegar. Put the bag on the head (like a chef's hat) and tie it in place with a long scarf. The headache should be relieved in 45 minutes.

Those plagued with nighttime leg cramps can find relief by supplementing meals with a glass of water, fortified with apple cider vinegar.

Prevent leg cramps by combining 1 teaspoon honey, 1 teaspoon apple cider vinegar, and 1 tablespoon calcium lactate in 1/2 glass of water. This is taken once a day.

Soothe tired or sprained muscles by wrapping the afflicted area with a cloth wrung out of apple cider vinegar. Leave it on for 3 to 5 minutes and repeat as needed. For extra special relief, add a good dash of cayenne pepper to the vinegar.

Banish the discomfort of nausea or vomiting by placing a cloth wrung out of warm apple cider vinegar on the stomach. Replace with another warm cloth when it cools.

You may ease the rasping of the evening cough by sleeping with the head on a cloth that has been steeped in vinegar.

An aching throat will be eased by rinsing it with water that has been made to blush by the addition of vinegar.

Difficult breathing may be eased by wrapping strips of white cloth, well dampened with vinegar, around the wrists.

Purify the waters of the body by sipping a tonic of goodly vinegar, mixed with clear running water.

Those who sup regularly of the miraculous vinegar will be

blessed with a sharp mind for all their life.

Bumps, lumps, and knots of the flesh may be relieved by the timely application of a binding soaked in the best vinegar.

Itching of the flesh may be relieved by the frequent application of vinegar.

Alleviate the discomfort of aching in the lower limbs by wrapping the afflicted area with a cloth wrung out of apple cider vinegar. When the binding begins to dry, renew it with fresh vinegar.

Folklore has long used vinegar for healing.

Make the suffering of one who speweth up their food less grievous by covering the belly with a well washed cloth, well soaked in warm vinegar.

ORAL TOLERATION

For many years doctors could find no reason to believe in the arthritis folk remedy that combines apple cider vinegar and honey in a daily tonic. New studies of how foods react in the body in a process called oral toleration may explain why this seems to work for some people. Vinegar's wide assortment of enzymes and amino acids may eventually be shown to desensitize the body to arthritis causing allergens. Perhaps one day soon foods will be considered preventive medicines, or even cures, for most degenerative diseases.

Consider using honey-sweetened vegetable or fruit fortified vinegar as a replacement for the time honored apple cider vinegar and honey arthritis remedy. It contains all the goodness of the original, combined with added nutritional benefits.

If oral toleration proves to be an answer to degenerative diseases, fortified vinegars will be an exceptional way to concentrate the benefits of many vegetables into one daily tonic.

ARTHRITIS & ALLERGIES

Food allergies can cause a feeling of extreme fatigue after meals. Foods can also cause bloating, congestion, itching, cramping, headaches and mood swings. Food sensitivity, a less dramatic reaction, has been linked to fatigue and joint pain.

The existence of allergic arthritis shows how very much food affects the immune system. Researchers are constantly adding to the medical community's knowledge of how food allergies can cause the body to produce chemicals that trigger inflammatory reactions. Those with arthritis may be particularly susceptible to food reactions because their immune systems already react in inappropriate ways. Zinc, magnesium, copper, vitamin B-6 and folic acid help regulate the immune system and may also minimize the side effects of anti-arthritis drugs. Many seasonings do more than make foods taste better. Arthritis pain may sometimes be eased by the actions of cayenne, ginger or turmeric.

No, hot foods such as cayenne peppers do not cause ulcers.

Foods affect the bacteria naturally present in the digestive system. Some have been linked to making rheumatoid arthritis symptoms worse. Mushrooms contain polysaccharides, complex carbohydrates that stimulate the body's natural immune response to both bacteria and viruses. They have been used for thousands of years in Eastern medicine to fight disease.

How Vinegar Has Been Used To Fight Disease

*W*hatever unpleasantness the body is exposed to, whether it is a harmful virus, deadly poison, infectious bacteria or damaging pollution, flavored acetic acid - that stuff we call vinegar - is involved in neutralizing it. Because it is a building block for living tissue plants, animals and humans need it. The body uses this natural by-product of healthy metabolism in many ways, including the manufacture of essential amino acids. It affects the way energy is released from fats and carbohydrates, and even how the body manufactures fat. Without its action the body could not make the life-giving red blood that delivers oxygen to the brain. When scientists examined molecules of glycogen, the body's sugar, they found it there, too.

When scientific research looks at old-time vinegar-based home remedies they have often been surprised to find many really work! Grandmother may not have been able to explain why her old remedies worked but she knew they did. Traditional Chinese Medicine (TCM), the system that has governed the health and long life of millions of

Chinese for thousands of years, without modern drugs, recognizes the value of vinegar. For example, TCM says those who regularly inhale the pleasant odor of vinegar have fewer problems with respiratory infections and more resistance to flu germs.

The body uses the acid we know as vinegar as a detoxifying agent. Molecules of this amazing liquid are able to connect themselves to many dangerous substances, including some drugs and poisons. This action creates entirely new compounds, which tend to be biologically inactive. Then, the body can safely expel these harmless substances.

A HEALING REMEDY – REDISCOVERED

Vinegar has always been around, but over the past few years sales of this miraculous food have increased dramatically. Flavored and organically pure varieties are now available in most grocery stores. As demand grows, more and more people are becoming aware of both its ability to improve the taste of foods and of its healthfulness.

One of biggest jobs vinegar does in the human body is to promote the growth of beneficial bacteria needed to keep disease-producing germs at bay. For example, human intestines contain millions of good bacteria (such as bifidus and lactobicillus) to keep the gastrointestinal tract healthy and disease free. Helpful bacteria in the intestines also:

- Support the immune system.
- Help digest food.
- Make some vitamins.
- Keep the intestines acidic.
- Discourage illness caused by E. coli and clostridia bacteria.

Phytochemicals are not vitamins. They are substances some researchers believe can actually change cancer cells back into normal ones. The National Cancer Institute is funding research, right now, to study phytochemicals. These seemingly magical chemicals can be frozen and microwaved and still heal. They are plentiful in both garlic and tomatoes, and very complex - there are estimated to be 10,000 different phytochemicals just in tomatoes.

Because isolating the action of a specific phytochemical is so difficult, it is best to eat whole vegetables. Pills and extracts will, almost certainly, not contain all the goodness of the complete food. A fortified vinegar that takes advantage of the many benefits of phytochemicals can be made by mixing 1 cup fresh tomato, 6 peeled garlic cloves and 1/2 cup apple cider vinegar in a blender. Some of the reasons to use this fortified vinegar are:

It contains compounds to thin the blood, prevent clotting and lower cholesterol and blood pressure.

Chemicals in it can stimulate release of the brain's natural tranquilizer, serotonin. It also can slow degeneration of brain cells. Some of these foods are used in China to improve senile dementia.

Sulfur based compounds in this vinegar have been shown to prevent the spread of some breast cancers.

Substances in it are believed to inhibit the spread of colon cancer.

This mix has ingredients that fight esophageal cancer.

Skin cancer has been shown to be inhibited by chemicals in these foods.

Many scientists believe substances in this fortified vinegar deter the spread of prostate cancers. (The chemicals that are so abundant in this mix of foods have actually killed some kinds of cancer cells.)

Strawberries, too, are being shown to have chemicals in them that fight cancer. They contain a polyphenol, called ellagic acid, which neutralizes carcinogens before they do their damage by invading DNA. And, it is thought strawberries interfere with the formation of nitrosamine in the intestines. (Nitrosamine can be very carcinogenic.) Make a vinegar which is strengthened with strawberries by combining in a blender: 1 cup strawberries, 1/2 cup apple cider vinegar, 1/4 cup honey.

Cranberries are another fruit that supplies the health benefits of ellagic acid. Serve them with vinegar and honey, too.

Ellagic acid in blackberries is not destroyed when it is cooked, so vinegar made with them can be used on grilled foods.

Fruit and honey vinegars fight breast cancer because they have lots of vitamin A.

Use sweet fruit-enhanced vinegars with a bit of brewer's yeast added to increase the amount of naturally occurring folate to deter colon cancer.

Once it was thought good nutrition was only important for babies and growing children. Now we realize the adult body needs adequate amounts of protein, carbohydrates, vitamins, minerals — as well as hundreds of trace elements — to function properly and to retard premature aging. The best mix of these substances, and sometimes the only place they can be found, is in the foods supplied to the body. We now know that, for adults, fruits and vegetables are more important than ever! Yet, dietitians tell us it is almost impossible to get all needed nutrients from the foods most people eat. If the diet does not contain enough leafy green vegetables, the body may be short of the folic acid needed to protect it from heart attack and stroke. A shortage of a tiny amount of a trace element can affect the emotions. If vitamin E, such as is found in wheat germ is in short supply, the risk of developing Parkinson's and Alzheimer's diseases may rise. The selenium in foods such as garlic help fight cancer and the beta carotene in cantaloupe and carrots is an antioxidant that soaks up free radicals that age the body.

Anti-oxidants in vegetables + fruits attack free radicals.

Free radical particles are left over from food digestion. These oxygen-rich substances damage body cells in the same way they make iron rust, vegetables rot and oils rancid. Free radicals can cause cells to lose their ability to function properly, or even die. Antioxidants such as flavonoids, carotenoids, vitamin C and vitamin E are the body's defense against free radicals. These protectives are found in fruits and vegetables. I have found that some very special things happen when lots of fruits and vegetables are added to the diet. They include:

A daily dose of pectin (the amount found in 2 or 3 apples) may be able to lower cholesterol — by as much as 25% or more.

Even when a diet contains more fat than doctors feel is healthy, extra fruits and vegetables can help lower blood pressure. And the benefits begin in as little as two weeks!

Adding garlic to the diet can reduce the likelihood of getting an infection. It fights 17 different kinds of fungus.

Eating lots of both garlic and onion has been linked to lower levels of cholesterol.

The carotenoid in tomatoes has twice the antioxidant power of beta carotene!

BETTER HEALTH WITH VINEGAR

For many years doctors could find no reason to believe in the arthritis folk remedy that combines apple cider vinegar and honey in a daily tonic. New studies of how foods react in the body in a process called oral toleration may explain why this seems to work for some people. Vinegar's wide assortment of enzymes and amino acids may eventually be shown to desensitize the body to arthritis causing allergens. Perhaps one day soon foods will be considered preventive medicines, or even cures, for most degenerative diseases. If oral toleration proves to be an answer to degenerative diseases, fortified vinegars will be an exceptional way to concentrate the benefits of many vegetables into one daily tonic.

Consider using honey-sweetened vegetable or fruit fortified vinegar as a replacement for the time honored apple cider vinegar and honey arthritis remedy. It contains all the goodness of the original, combined with added nutritional benefits.

FIGHT GERMS

To relieve the pain of a sore throat caused by a cold, mix together 1/4 cup honey and 1/4 cup apple cider vinegar. Take 1 tablespoon every 4 hours. May be taken more often if needed.

Ease the discomfort of a sore throat and speed healing by sipping occasionally on a syrup made of 1/2 cup apple cider vinegar, 1/2 cup water, 1 teaspoon cayenne pepper, and 3 tablespoons honey.

A vinegar gargle can ease the pain of a sore throat. Just gargle with a glass of warm water to which a tablespoon of apple cider vinegar has been added. Repeat as needed. This also acts as a great mouthwash!

Soothe a dry night cough by sprinkling the pillowcase with apple cider vinegar.

A small amount of vinegar, taken every day, keeps the urinary tract nice and acidy. This is useful to reduce the likelihood of getting a kidney or bladder infection.

To chase away a cold, soak an eight-inch square of brown paper (cut from a paper grocery bag) in apple cider vinegar. When the paper is saturated, sprinkle it with pepper and bind to the chest with cloth strips, pepper side of the paper next to the skin. After 20 minutes, remove the paper and wash the chest, being careful not to become chilled.

If troubled by the itching and peeling of athlete's foot, soak socks or hose in vinegar water. Mix 1 part vinegar with 5 parts water and soak them for 30 minutes before washing as usual.

Asthma can be relieved by combining the advantages of acupressure with the benefits of apple cider vinegar. Use a wide rubber band to hold gauze pads, which have been soaked in vinegar, to the inside of the wrists.

VINEGAR FIGHTS DISEASE

Apple cider vinegar enthusiasts can recite a long list of ailments it is reported to be able to cure or prevent. It is claimed vinegar can banish arthritis, forestall osteoporosis, prevent cancer, kill infection, condition the skin, aid digestion, control weight, preserve memory, and protect the mind from aging. On the pages which follow some of the most recent findings of medical researchers, and the way this research impacts on vinegar therapy, are recorded. Also included are some of the more enduring traditional remedies.

One reason apple cider vinegar seems to do so much of what is claimed for it is because it contains such a marvelous combination of tart good taste and germ killing acids. Vinegar is fermented from sweet apple cider, and takes its honey-gold color from tannins that flow from ruptured cell walls of fresh, ripe apples. When these naturally occurring, colorless preservatives, come into contact with air they develop the rich, golden color we associate with cider. This is called enzymatic browning. It contributes to the distinctive flavor of cider, a flavor with more spunk than simple apple juice.

Please remember, if you have a specific illness, or take medication regularly, discuss the effects of adding vinegar to your diet with your doctor.

More recently, vinegar has been used to treat chronic middle ear diseases when traditional drug-based methods fail. One treatment currently being prescribed for ear infections at Ohio State University's hospital is irrigation with vinegar.

Vinegar is at home in the hospital.

37

Doctors are currently considering the possibility of treating some eye infections with diluted vinegar. Right now, they are using it as a hospital disinfectant. One example of this use is at Yale-New Haven Hospital. When after-surgery eye infections became a problem, their Department of Bacteriology solved the problem with common vinegar. The hospital began routinely cleaning the scrub-room sink with a 1/2% solution of ordinary household vinegar. It worked better at elimination the offending bacteria than the commercial product it replaced!

EARS

Grandmother said putting diluted vinegar in the ears would ward off infection. Now medical authorities have confirmed her wisdom. The American Academy of Otolaryngology (head and neck surgery) suggests using a mixture of vinegar and alcohol to prevent swimmer's ear. Infections, as well as plain old itchy ears, are a common compliant of swimmers. Doctors specializing in treating these ailments now recommend using vinegar as a preventive. Simply dilute vinegar half and half with boiled water and use to rinse out the ears after each swim. For a more drying solution, mix vinegar half and half with alcohol. This helps to prevent both bacterial and fungus growths.
Never self treat ear infections! Improperly treated ear infections can rapidly turn into very serious illness, especially in little ones!

SKIN AILMENTS

Two old-time remedies for treating mild burns were to douse the hurt with apple cider vinegar or to let a snail crawl over it. If you don't have a friendly snail around, you may want to try dabbing a bit of apple cider vinegar onto the painful area. Vinegar is particularly useful for neutralizing alkali burns.

Relieve itchy skin, too, by patting on apple cider vinegar. If the itch is near the eyes or other delicate areas dilute the vinegar, 4 parts water to 1 part vinegar. For a full body treatment, put 2 or 3 cups in the bath water. A handful of thyme can help, too.

Dampen a gauze square in apple cider vinegar and apply, gently, ease to rectal itching.

Rashes caused by infections may be made to go away by nibbling on the mother that floats on a good vinegar.

VINEGAR AND DIGESTION

Apple cider vinegar is very similar to the chemicals found naturally in the stomach. Because of this, it has traditionally been hailed as an aid to digestion. And so, by improving digestion, it is felt it will improve the overall metabolism of the body.

Those who regularly imbibe of this elixir feel it helps cuts and abrasions heal faster, as well as speeding up the healing of more serious wounds.

Vinegar is considered by many to be able to attack and kill harmful bacteria which has invaded the digestive tract. This may lessen the likelihood of the body developing toxemia and other blood-borne infections.

Some doctors suggest regular vinegar use to prevent food poisoning. They recommend its use when visiting questionable restaurants or foreign countries. The usual dose is to take 1 tablespoon of vinegar, 30 minutes before meals. It can be mixed with a glass of water, vegetable juice, or any other beverage. Honey added to vinegar and water makes the taste more palatable for most people.

A vinegar experiment anyone can try is to use it to make legumes more digestible, and so less gas producing. Just splash a little vinegar in the pot when cooking dried beans. It will make them tender and easy on the digestive system.

CANCER, VINEGAR AND BETA CAROTENE

Aging, heart disease, cancer, and cataracts are symptoms of the harm done to the human body by free radicals, the "loose cannons" of the cell world. They damage chromosomes and are probably responsible for many of the physical changes associated with aging.

Free radicals roam through plants, animals, and humans, bouncing from cell to cell, damaging each in turn. Antioxidants absorb free radicals, making them harmless. Beta carotene, a carotenoid found in vinegar, is a powerful antioxidant.

Carotenoids probably protect plants from solar radiation.

Carotenoid occurs naturally in plants such as apples. Vinegar's beta carotene is in a natural, easy to digest form. One example of how this antioxidant contributes to maintaining good health is the way it protects the eye from cataracts. Cataract development is related to oxidation of the eye's lens. This happens when free radicals alter its structure. Studies show that eating lots of antioxidant containing foods decreases the risk of forming cataracts.

A correlation between eating lots of beta carotene containing foods and a lower risk of cancer has also been documented. Researchers, in more than 70 different studies, agree beta carotene lowers the risk of getting cancer. They include those at the State University of New York at Stony Brook, the University of Western Ontario in Canada, Tufts University, and Johns Hopkins School of Medicine.

In addition to giving cancer protection, beta carotene boosts the body's immune system. It works by attacking the free radicals which destroy the immune system.

Carotenoids are also the body's raw material for producing vitamin A, another potent antioxidant. They act together to protect from cancers associated with chemical toxins. According to National Cancer Research in England, when the body does not get enough vitamin A, it is particularly susceptible to cancers of the respiratory system, bladder and colon.

Vinegar fights cancer by inhibiting glycolysis.

Old timers have long recommended taking a teaspoon of vinegar, every day, in a tall glass of vegetable juice. With all we now know about fiber and beta carotene, this may turn out to be very good advice!

More than half of women's cancers can be traced to diet. Breasts seem to be particularly sensitive to food toxins such as pesticides and partially hydrogenated oil preservatives. This is probably because these oil soluble chemicals tend to be stored in breast fat. Lower the risk of breast cancer by eating soy products for their phytoestrogens (plant estrogens). Eat broccoli, cauliflower and kale for their effect on the way the body uses estrogen.

Garlic is considered an anti-cancer food because it stops the activity of some substances which are known to cause cancer. It seems to work on both existing cancers and as a preventive against new ones. Garlic lowers the risk of developing many diseases because it strengthens the immune system.

CANCER DETECTION

Western Michigan University reports early test results which indicate vinegar can be used to increase the accuracy of conventional tests for cervical cancer. Adding the new vinegar-based test to the standard test allows medical personnel to "...detect women at risk for cervical cancer who would not have been detected by the Pap test alone." The vinegar test simple for technicians, low-cost, non-invasive, and safe for the patient.

Scientists at the A.P. John Institute for Cancer Research recently announced that they are adding vinegar supplements to the diets of their patients because they feel it helps in "…. Shutting off cancer cells energy supply and causing them to die off."

VINEGAR & ARTHRITIS

50 years ago a daily apple cider vinegar and honey tonic was recommended to ease arthritis. During the past 30 years, "wonder drugs" have replaced it and other folk remedies. Now, vinegar and many other old-time remedies are finding new followers, including many medical professionals. One reason for vinegar's renewed appeal is that almost everyone has experienced the negative side effects of today's powerful new drugs. Apple cider vinegar's double fermentation results in an assortment of enzymes and amino acids whose combined actions are not completely understood by researchers. It is very possible this old remedy will, one day soon, be shown to desensitize the body to arthritis causing allergens as it strengthens the immune system. The immune system and arthritis have very strong ties. It mediates the body's power to heal and repair itself. A weak immune system does not aggressively repair cell damage. And, an undernourished immune system cannot tell the difference between invading germs and healthy body tissue. So, it attacks and destroys cartilage in joints. It also loses the ability to lay down as much new cartilage in joints as is worn away.

Eat a variety of colors, each day.

SUNBURN & CAROTENOIDS

Carotenoids, those amazing substances in vegetables and fruits, can reduce sunburn damage by UV rays! New research indicates eating carotenoid rich vegetables and fruits can also be a preventive against skin cancer. It has been suggested that supplements of carotenoids, taken before going out in the sun, may be as effective as sun screens. This is

41

another reason to use fortified vinegars to increase the amount of these foods in your diet!

Each carotenoid seems to protect a particular part of the body or type of cell. They also have different ways of providing this antioxidant protection. Some foods, and what they contain follow:

Cantaloupe, carrots, pumpkin	alpha carotene
Apricots, carrots, sweet potatoes	beta carotene
Oranges, peaches, tangerines	beta-cryptoxanthin
Apricots, tomatoes	gamma carotene
Red peppers, mustard greens	lutein
Tomatoes, watermelon	lycopene
Beet tops, kale	zeaxanthin

ILLNESS & DIET

General aging of the brain has been linked to damage caused by free radicals. Specifically, confusion and memory loss can be caused by too little vitamin B-12 or folic acid. Some depression is associated with a deficiency of folic acid, calcium, iron, copper, magnesium or potassium. Macular degeneration is fought by the lutein and zeaxanthin in kale, spinach and several kinds of peppers.

Dark green and orange vegetables are rich in carotenoids that the body converts to vitamin A. It is needed by the body to make rhodopsin. This substance is essential to night vision and helps cut the risk of developing macular degeneration, one of the most common causes of blindness.

Prostate, breast and endometrial cancers seem to be restrained by lycopene. It is a carotenoid in tomatoes, pink grapefruit, apricots and watermelon.

Calcium loss from bones and menopause symptoms can both be reduced by estrogen-like isoflavones in soybeans. Psoriasis is less common in those who eat lots of fresh fruit, carrots and tomatoes.

Doctors are searching for better ways to fight deadly infections, such as tuberculosis, with diet changes. Perhaps one day they will confirm the existence of specific foods that have the ability to regulate the immune system. In the meantime, most recommend a low saturated fat regimen that features lots of vegetables and fruits and a minimum of animal protein.

MORE MOTHER-OF-VINEGAR USES

Not everyone finds mother appealing.

While mother of vinegar may not seem to many to be a particularly appetizing snack, some claim it is endowed with nearly miraculous healing properties. Some old-time mother-of-vinegar remedies follow:

Dip out a goodly spoonful of the moldy mother-of-vinegar from the top of a vinegar barrel and eat it very slowly. This healthy slime will relieve joint pains and headaches caused by infections.

A bit of mother-of-vinegar, taken each day, prevents most infectious diseases.

Scoop the stringy mass of mother-of-vinegar from the bottom of a barrel that has held vinegar and save it for treating infectious diseases. Preserve it by mixing it half and half with honey. One small teaspoon of this honey and mother mixture, taken twice a day, gives protection from infectious diseases and parasite infestation.

Take a bite or two of mother-of-vinegar, morning and evening. It will keep grievous germs and nasty parasites away from the body.

Grow your own mother-of-vinegar, to hurry along homemade vinegar, or for nibbling, by combining 1 cup of vinegar and 1 cup of fresh cider. Let this set, open to the air, for a few days (or weeks, depending on the temperature). The scum that forms on the surface is mother-of-vinegar.

UN – CLOGGING ARTERIES

"Coronary artery disease can be stopped in its tracks, even reversed, without drugs!" That is what researchers say about an eating plan very much like the vinegar diet. Their studies suggest the nutrients found in abundance in vegetables and fruits can improve the condition of arteries. Nutrition therapy can help even if there are no obvious signs of deficiencies. Extra amounts of vitamin C, chromium, magnesium, selenium, niacin and potassium are especially helpful.

New studies report those who eat a salad every day have fewer heart attacks. When eggplant is eaten with foods high in vitamin C it seems to protect the body from developing fatty plaques in the arteries. Vegetables are excellent foods, but they do not take the place of fruits.

43

Eating both fresh fruits and vegetables, every day, has been linked to a significant reduction in fatal heart attacks and strokes.

Ginger is very good for artery health. It helps lower cholesterol and seems to discourage cells from sticking together to form clots.

FIBER

A low fat, high fiber diet helps deter heart attacks, strokes and cancer. One way fiber fights cancer is by quickly pushing toxin laden food through the colon. Fiber helps reduce the likelihood of developing stomach ulcers because food and its digestive acids spend less time in the body. Its bulk eases constipation and its water absorbing capabilities moderates diarrhea. Soluble fiber in legumes such as pinto, navy, kidney and soy beans protects good HDL cholesterol and lowers bad LDL. They begin their cholesterol lowering work almost immediately.

Fiber, particularly the soluble fiber in foods like oatmeal, helps remove cholesterol from the body. Too much fiber, such as is in some supplements can interfere with calcium absorption.

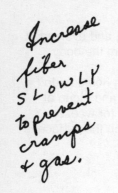
Increase fiber SLOWLY to prevent cramps & gas.

The membrane holding together sections of grapefruit is an especially healthy fiber. Half of it is soluble to soak up cholesterol, half is insoluble to fight constipation and colon cancer. Two grapefruit have a full day's fiber needs.

Vinegars fortified with apples or sweet potatoes are high fiber foods that can help ease hemorrhoids.

Diabetes is at least as deadly for adult women as breast cancer! A high fiber, low fat, diet and exercise are the recommended preventatives.

FAT

All fuels produce by-products when they are burned. Some of these by-products are more harmful than others. Foods high in saturated fats produce more toxic chemicals than vegetables, fruits and whole grains. Some fat is necessary for good health, even the body makes a bit of cholesterol.

The healthiest diet seems to be one with a small amount of the right kinds of oil added to it. Polyunsaturated oils such as flaxseed, corn, safflower and soy are good for use in cold dishes. Flaxseed is a rich source of the omega-3 oils also found in cold water fish. But when polyunsaturated oils are heated they produce toxic lipid peroxides. So, for cooking, the oleic acid containing monounsaturated oils are best. Two good heat and light resistant monounsaturated oils are olive and canola.

Fat substitutes are used in many processed foods. Simplesse® is one that has been used for many years. Avicel® is a cellulose gel. N-Oil® is a tapioca based dextrin. Olestra®, one of the newest fat substitutes, is calorie free, but may inhibit fat soluble vitamins such as A, D, E and K. It may also interfere with the absorption of important carotenoids.

FOOD & CHEMO-PREVENTIVES

Turmeric is a very safe, anti-UV radiation antioxidant. It has even been shown to help prevent chromosome damage.

Rosemary contains substances that act against free radicals. It also protects the liver from the damage that can be done by some toxins. Rosemary's phenolic compounds, carnosol and carnosic acid do this antioxidant work. These flavonoids can be used as preservatives for fats in foods.

Ginger has substances to help protect the liver. It is also useful against platelet clumping, which contributes to heart attacks. Apples, onions and tea contain flavonoids, antioxidants to reduce the risk of heart disease.

Garlic has substances that energize the immune system. One of these, selenium, has been found to lower the risk of cancer of the colon, lung, prostate and rectal.

Carotenoids, those amazing substances in vegetables and fruits, can help limit the spread of breast cancer. Tests are being conducted on using them to stop the spread of lung, stomach and colon cancers, too. Beta carotene helps maintain healthy eyes. When taken at the same time as aspirin, it may prevent some side effects, such as stomach distress.

Vinegar Does A Body Good Feel Young, Look Good

So you want to live forever! Apple cider vinegar contains the healthy goodness of apples, concentrated into a teaspoon of golden liquid. It is packed with essential amino acids and healthful enzymes. And so it comes as no surprise that some individuals have claimed this natural storehouse of vitamins and minerals will cure all that ails mankind -- and even extend life and youthfulness.

Is apple cider vinegar an instant remedy for all the ills of this world? A magical nostrum? A mystical elixir? A liquid cure all? Some believe it is something very close to this!

Traditional medical systems are sickness oriented, in that they are designed to respond to illness. But good health, and extending life's best years begins with a body that is maintained every day by good eating and health practices. A healthy, ageless body requires a diet rich in a wide assortment of nutrients. And the safest way to get adequate nutrients is to supply the body with a varied diet. It should meet all known nutritional requirements and be enhanced with lots of trace elements.

Perhaps this is why apple cider vinegar has the reputation of being an almost magical tonic -- one of the most healthful, nutrient filled fluids known to mankind. A teaspoon of this golden liquid supplies a generous portion of the building blocks needed to be a healthy being. This potent substance is endowed with a multitude of vitamins, minerals and essential amino acids.

Scientists know humans need very tiny amounts of hundreds of as yet largely unidentified compounds. Nutritional researchers are constantly discovering minerals, enzymes, amino acids, and other substances and essences the body needs for complete health. Exactly how the body uses trace elements remains a medical mystery. Nor has science identified the amount needed of most of them.

I have the feeling vinegar has been around as long as apples!

Doctors do know a tiny deficiency, a missing milli-microgram of an important element can result in sickness, premature aging or damage to the mind. The best advice nutritional scientists can give is to eat a diet of assorted foods, making a broad spectrum of nutrients available to the body.

Since the beginning of time mankind has sought the magic elixir that bubbles from the fabled Fountain of Youth. For most of us, apple cider vinegar may be as close as we will ever come to such a universal remedy. Because, you see, the secret to eternal youth is already ours. It is simply to be vital and able to enjoy a zestful, vigorous, life every single day we live.

So, it is no wonder apple cider vinegar is a time-honored prescription for those who want to retain vitality and good health well into old age. Through the ages it has been prescribed as an aid in maintaining general health, preventing disease, controlling weight, easing the discomfort of coughs, colds and breathing difficulties, and settling a disturbed digestive system.

Because old-time remedies (such as those in this book) are handed down from parent to child to grandchild, over many generations, changes occur. Families develop their own variations. Yet, there is one constant theme: some small amount of apple cider vinegar, taken each day, somehow brings better health and longer life. Folklore recommends these ways to live a long, healthy, vital life:

Ensure long life and health by drinking vinegar every day. Simply add a tablespoon to a full glass of water and drink it down.

Memory can be greatly improved by drinking a glass of warm water before each meal, with a teaspoon of apple cider vinegar stirred in.

The way to stay healthy and alert, well into old age, is to combine 1 teaspoon of vinegar, 1 teaspoon of honey, and a full glass of water. Take this tonic 3 times a day, 1/2 hour before meals.

For a long, vigorous life, filled with robust good health, sip a vinegar tonic, very slowly, before each meal. Mix together and begin drinking immediately: 1 cup warm water, 2 tablespoons apple cider vinegar, and 1 teaspoon honey.

The most palatable way to take a daily dose of vinegar is to add a small dollop of clover honey to a tablespoon of vinegar and a teaspoon of olive oil. Mix it all together and drip this healthy dressing over a small bowl of greens.

A health promoting salad dressing can be made from 1/4 cup vinegar, 1/4 cup corn oil, and 1/8 cup honey. Mix well and serve at the evening meal to keep the whole family in good health.

Feel Young, Look Good

Much of the body's aging is caused by free radicals. They occur naturally as a by-product of metabolism and are responsible for the degenerative diseases we call aging. Free radicals weaken the immune system, cause the skin to wrinkle and accelerate the development of arthritis. Antioxidants are the body's defense against free radicals. Primary antioxidants are natural (or synthetic) chemicals that contain either a phenol ring, or a chemical equivalent. In addition to esters formed by fermentation, vinegar picks up phenols from wood during its manufacture and while stored in wood barrels. Secondary antioxidants are usually acids; 4% to 6% acetic acid is the basis for all vinegar. Free radicals are especially devastating to the lipids which form cell membranes.

Grandmother used vinegar for good health.

When free radicals attack, cells collapse and the skin forms wrinkles. Beta carotene, selenium and vitamins C and E are some of the strongest antioxidants. When vinegar is infused with powerful antioxidant containing herbs it takes on their qualities, while retaining its own. This kind of antioxidant supplementation has many advantages over pills because when only one chemical is added to the body it can cause an imbalance that

48

destroys or depletes others.

Specialty vinegars taste good and heal the body. They offer a way to add nutrients in a balanced way, by increasing wholesome foods in the diet. Creamy vinegars can add significant amounts of beta-carotene and vegetable flavorids to food. Clear vinegars leach vitamins, minerals and trace elements from herbs soaked in it. These antioxidants help the body repair the damage done by free radicals. Make clear herb vinegars by adding a few fresh sprigs or a tablespoon of dried herb to a bottle of vinegar. Let set for 3 or 4 weeks and strain. Use on salads, boiled pastas or meats. The vinegars that follow are especially good to fight aging by strengthening the immune system:

Marjoram helps the body fight inflammation and is especially good at reducing the effects of lung infections. Use leaves and flowers.

Columbine has trigloquinine to calm the mind and ease gastrointestinal disorders.

Peppermint leaves contain several healthful flavonoids, including xanthomicrol and luteolin glycoside. This vinegar is good on greens and meats, as well as being a mood enhancing aerosol.

A small sliver of ginseng root, soaked in a bottle of vinegar for a few weeks, produces a tonic to invigorate the body and mind. Ginseng has been used to deter aging for many centuries.

Goldenseal root produces a vinegar for healing infections and contagious diseases.

Make a thick, antioxidant fortified vinegar to serve over fresh greens, cooked vegetables, pasta or fruits by combining a cup of apple cider vinegar with half a dozen peeled garlic cloves and a cup each of broccoli, spinach, sweet potato and onion in a blender.

Red clover makes a pretty vinegar that some believe can help the body fight cancer, as well as many degenerative diseases.

Licorice root has been found to stimulate the body's ability to produce interferon. This makes it important in fighting all diseases that prey on a weak immune system.

Rosemary adds calcium, magnesium, phosphorus, potassium and other minerals that both the nerves and heart muscle need to function properly.

Black cohosh has been shown to be an excellent herb for strengthening the vascular system. It is also considered a central nervous system tonic and a muscle relaxant.

Passion flower contains both flavenoids and glycosides. This herb has been used for hundreds of years to calm and soothe nervous tension.

A piece of the root of the common burdock makes a vinegar that helps the body recover from disease. It may also help prevent sickness.

LOOK BETTER, FEEL BETTER

Vinegar which has been made even better by adding other ingredients to it is also good for the outside of the body. Some ways to use vinegar for smooth, young looking skin and bright, shining hair follow:

The most marvelous tonic for the feet is to walk back and forth in ankle deep bath water to which 1/2 cup apple cider vinegar has been added. Do this for 5 minutes, first thing in the morning, and for 5 minutes before retiring in the evening. Hot, aching feet will feel cooled and soothed.

A full head of healthy, richly colored hair can be ensured, well into old age. You need only to start each day with a glass of water to which has been added 4 teaspoons each of apple cider vinegar, black strap molasses, and honey.

Heavily soiled hands can be cleaned while giving them a soothing treatment. Simply scrub with cornmeal, moistened with apple cider vinegar. Then rinse in cool water and pat dry.

You can banish dandruff and make hair shiny and healthy if you rinse after every shampoo with 1/2 cup apple cider vinegar mixed into two cups of warm water. It also brightens dark hair and adds sparkle to blond hair.

Ensure soft, radiant skin and prevent blemishes by conditioning the skin while sleeping with a covering of strawberries and vinegar. Mash 3 large strawberries into 1/4 cup vinegar and let it sit for 2 hours. Then strain the vinegar through a cloth. Pat the strawberry infused vinegar onto the face and neck and leave on until morning. Skin will soon be free of pimples and blackheads.

Corns and calluses will fall away, overnight, if you treat them with a vinegar compress. Simply tape 1/2 of a slice of stale bread (which has been soaked with apple cider vinegar) to the offending lump. By morning the skin will look smooth and new.

Ladies can protect their skin from the ravages of the summer sun by applying a protective of olive oil and apple cider vinegar. Mixed half and half, this combination helps prevent sunburn and chapping.

Age spots can be gotten rid of if you wipe them daily with onion juice and vinegar. Mix together 1 teaspoon onion juice and 2 teaspoons vinegar and apply with a soft cloth. Or, 1/2 a fresh onion can be dipped into a small dish of vinegar and then rubbed across the offending skin. In a few weeks the spot will begin to fade.

Age spots are sometimes called liver spots.

Itchy welts and hives, swellings and blemishes can be eased by the application of a paste made from vinegar and cornstarch. Just pat it on and feel the itch being drawn out as the paste dries.

Relieve the discomfort and unsightliness of varicose veins by wrapping the legs with a cloth wrung out of apple cider vinegar. Leave this on, with the legs propped up, for 30 minutes morning and evening. Considerable relief will be noticed within a few weeks. To speed up the healing process, follow each treatment with a glass of warm water, to which a teaspoon of apple cider vinegar has been added. Sip slowly, and add a teaspoon of honey if feeling over-tired.

Use a cloth moistened in vinegar to clean armpits. Do not rinse it off and it will eliminate offensive odors for several hours.

Cool the burning of a sunburn by bathing in a tub of lukewarm water, to which a cup of apple cider vinegar has been added. Whenever a sprain or ache needs to be soaked in very hot water, a splash of vinegar in the water will make the water seem cooler.

One reason vinegar is so very helpful in treating skin disorders is that it has a pH which is nearly the same as healthy skin. So, applying vinegar helps to normalize the pH of the skin's surface.

ESPECIALLY FOR WOMEN

Vinegar Facial Mask
1/4 cup oatmeal
 1 tablespoon honey
 1 tablespoon apple cider vinegar
    Combine ingredients and pat the mixture onto wet skin. Let set until dry. Wash off with cool water and apply moisturizer.

Skin Soothing Bath
    Put 1 cup vegetable oil in a bottle and add 1/4 cup apple cider vinegar and 2 tablespoons liquid hand soap. Shake well before adding a few cupfuls to bath water. A few drops of perfume may be added, if desired. Or, replace the apple cider vinegar with lavender, rosemary or woodruff herbal vinegar.

Hair Moisturizer
 1 egg yolk
 1 teaspoon honey
1/4 cup olive oil
1/4 cup apple cider vinegar
    Beat all ingredients together for several minutes, or combine in a blender to produce a thick, smooth cream. Rub the mixture into the hair and onto the scalp and let set for about 10 minutes. Shampoo out and rinse in lukewarm water with a splash of apple cider vinegar added to it.

Skin Lightening Solution
1/4 cup white vinegar
1/4 cup lemon juice
 1 cup white wine
 1 tablespoon honey
    Put all ingredients into a jar and shake until will mixed. Pat onto the skin morning and evening.

Shiny Hair Spray
    Combine 1 cup water and 1/4 cup apple cider vinegar in a pump-spray bottle. A light spritz will add sparkling highlights and a bit of body to dull, limp hair. It works even better with a drop or two of perfume added to it, or if the apple cider vinegar is replaced with herbal vinegar.

Oil & Vinegar Hair Treatment
    Restore the health of dry, sun damaged hair with oil and vinegar! Heat 1/4 cup olive oil until it is comfortably warm and then massage it into the scalp and hair. Make sure ends get a good coating, using

extra oil for long hair. Next, add 1/2 cup apple cider vinegar to a sink full of very hot water. Soak a towel in the hot vinegar water and then wring it out. Wrap the warm, wet towel around the olive oil treated hair and cover with a second, dry towel. After 15 minutes, remove both towels and wash the hair with a gentle shampoo.

Wash this out before it dries

Soft Skin - Forever

Keep the skin on your face soft and youthful looking by moisturizing it before applying makeup. Just wring a washcloth out of warm water with a dash of vinegar in it. Hold the warm, wet washcloth over the face for 15 - 20 seconds, pat the skin barely dry, then apply moisturizer, followed by makeup. Skin will remain soft and youthful looking, and will be less likely to develop blemishes.

ESPECIALLY FOR MEN

Men's Scented Splash-On

Vinegar with spices and herbs added to it was the original skin tonic for men. Begin by mixing together a basic aftershave lotion of 1 cup white vinegar and 2 tablespoons sweet clover honey. Add 1 tablespoon of an aromatic herb. Let the preparation set for a week, strain out the herb leaves and the aftershave lotion is ready to use! Some especially fragrant herbs for aftershave lotions are sage, thyme, cloves, bay and coriander. Combine a couple of herbs to make your own distinctive scent. Some of the best ones for tightening and conditioning the skin are made with spearmint, bee balm, chamomile or blackberry leaves.

Skin Bracer

For a healing, refreshing facial tonic, mix 1/2 teaspoon cream of tartar and two tablespoons vinegar into a half cup of warm water. Pat onto the face after washing.

Aftershave

Combine 1/2 cup white vinegar, 1/2 cup vodka and 2 tablespoons honey. Spice it up by soaking 1 teaspoon aromatic herbs in the mixture for about a month, then strain and use. Apple cider vinegar, substituted for the white vinegar, makes a more robust aftershave. Rubbing alcohol may be substituted for the vodka for a less expensive version. A teaspoon of glycerin added to the aftershave mixture will soothe and moisturize a dry face.

53

Men deserve vinegar skin care, too.

Refrigerated Aftershave

This is a cooling aftershave for warm weather use. Puree a small cucumber in the blender (do not peel) with several fresh mint leaves. Add this mixture to a basic vinegar aftershave and set in the refrigerator overnight. Strain and it is ready to use. (Must be kept refrigerated.)

VINEGAR IS FOR PEOPLE

Over the years vinegar has been credited with the power to act as a soothing skin tonic, add shining highlights to hair and, when combined with herbs, bring calming comfort or energizing zest to the bath. What follows is a collection of old-fashioned remedies that use vinegar to make people feel better. Please remember, these old-time remedies are not medically proven. They are simply ways many people have used vinegar mixtures for relief of discomfort and for its fresh, pleasing aroma.

Instantly Soft Hands

Pour 1/2 cup water, with 1 teaspoon vinegar stirred in, over the hands. Sprinkle with 1/2 teaspoon white sugar, then with 1 teaspoon baby oil. Work this mixture into the hands for 2 minutes, then wash with a gentle soap. Hands will be almost magically smooth and velvety feeling!

Silky Smooth Hands

Add 1 tablespoon apple cider vinegar to 2 cups warm water. Soak hands in this mixture for 5 minutes, then pat them dry. Smooth 1/2 teaspoon petroleum jelly over the hands and pull on a pair of cotton gloves. By morning the hands will be unbelievably soft and smooth, no matter how much hard work they do during the day.

Soft Feet

Rough skin on the feet can be softened by soaking them in water and vinegar, then applying body lotion. Use lukewarm water, with a tablespoon of apple cider vinegar added for each quart of water. Pat the feet completely dry, gently apply body lotion, then cover with cotton socks.

Softer Feet

Hard, dry calluses and coarse skin can make feet feel uncomfortable, and contribute to pain when walking. Soften feet by soaking for 5 minutes in warm water with a little vinegar in it, then rubbing granulated white sugar over rough spots. Follow with a quick baby oil massage, then wash thoroughly with a gentle soap before covering with cotton socks. (Baby oil makes feet VERY slippery! Always wash it all off BEFORE standing or walking.)

Everyone needs a little Vinegar.

Soften Corns & Calluses

To soften skin made rough and scaly by corns and calluses, soak the feet every day in a pan of warm soapy water, to which a cup of vinegar has been added.

Foot Odor

Banish foot odor by soaking feet in strong tea. Follow with a rinse made from 1 cup warm water and 1 cup apple cider vinegar.

Easier Nail Trimming

If tough toenails make trimming them a chore, soak the feet in warm water with a couple of tablespoons of vinegar added to it. After about 10 minutes, nails will be much softer and easier to trim.

Steamy Vinegar Facial

Heat 1 cup herbal vinegar to the boiling point and pour it into a large bowl. Lean over the bowl and drape a towel over your head and the bowl. Allow the warm, moist steam to soften facial skin. When the vinegar has cooled, pat it onto the face as a cleansing astringent. Strawberry vinegar is especially good for the skin.

Nice Facial

Blend together 1/2 cup apple cider vinegar and 1/4 cup well-cooked rice and 1/4 cup cooked oatmeal. Spread this mixture on the face, neck and shoulders. Allow to dry for 10 minutes, then wash off and pat dry with a soft towel. Skin will be soft and smooth.

Better Facial

For a refining facial, combine 1 tablespoon apple cider vinegar, 1 tablespoon honey and 1/2 a mashed banana. Apply a generous coating and after five minutes your skin will feel revitalized. Strawberries or a peach may be used in place of the banana. Or, make a paste of dry yeast and warm water. Pat this onto the face and allow to dry. Rinse off with warm water. Then, rinse again with a quart of cool water to which a tablespoon of apple cider vinegar has been added.

Grandmother's Dandruff Treatment

After washing and rinsing the hair as usual, treat it to 5 minutes of conditioning with a mixture of 1/2 cup apple cider vinegar to which

2 aspirins have been added. Rinse well, then follow with a final conditioning rinse of a quart of warm water to which 1/2 cup apple cider vinegar has been added.

Herbal Baths

Homemade scented vinegars are the essential component of great herbal baths. Use 1/4 to 1/2 cup vinegar to a tub of warm water. For a relaxing soak, use herbal vinegars such as catnip, lemon balm, lavender, borage, chamomile or slippery elm. For an invigorating soak, use herbal vinegars such as ginger, peppermint, sage, or tarragon.

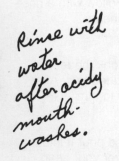
Rinse with water after acidy mouth-washes.

Flavorful Mouthwashes

A glass of water with a couple of teaspoons of vinegar in it is a traditional mouthwash and gargle liquid. Use white vinegar for a neutral taste, apple cider vinegar for its healing reputation, or herbal for breath enhancing flavor. Some good herbal vinegars for mouthwashes are sage, raspberry, peppermint and lavender.

Denture Cleaner and Freshener

A quick brushing with white vinegar will help to brighten dentures. It will also remove lingering odors. If dentures are set overnight in water, adding 1/2 teaspoon vinegar will help keep them odor free. Using apple cider vinegar will add a refreshing flavor to the mouth. Herbal vinegars, such as thyme or mint, also act as breath fresheners.

Nail Polish

Nail Polish will go on smoother, and stay on longer if you clean your fingernails with white vinegar before applying the polish.

Tonics And Elixirs For A Healthy Mind & Body

A loving heart, a sharp mind and a healthy body – these are signs of a successful life. Down through thousands of years folklore has tied reaching these goals to the use of vinegar in all its many forms. Many ways to use this wondrous fluid alone, or combined with other healthful foods follow. They integrate the latest findings of medical food researchers with the wisdom of traditional healing ways.

VINEGAR AND THE MIND

Memory loss is one of the most common and costly of the diseases whose frequency increases with age. Its price to this country approaches $50 billion a year. That, of course, is only the cost in dollars. The real cost is in disrupted families, shattered lives and unrelenting heartache. For those suffering with memory loss, quality of life is ruined and, often, it is ruined for their loved ones as well.

The three most common causes of memory loss are Alzheimer's disease, multiple strokes (multi-infarct dementia) and alcohol abuse. Increasingly, many other elders endure mental impairment caused by poor nutrition and reactions to prescription drugs.

Too often memory loss in individuals who are over 55 is treated as if it were irreversible or inevitable. Yet, information continues to pile up that indicates that many cases of memory loss can be successfully treated. More and more doctors are echoing the words of one specialist: "...several of the causes are treatable, resulting in an arrest or actual reversal of the symptoms."

Diet is an important factor in control of risk factors for memory loss, and to reverse damage that has already been done. Good nutrition can decrease the likelihood of mind crippling strokes by lowering cholesterol. It can also protect the mind from some of the worse causes of loss of mental function. *The Journal of the American Dietetic Association* puts it this way: "Some forms of dementia -- those due to excessive alcohol intake or vitamin deficiency -- may be entirely preventable and partially reversible through diet."

Dementia that is associated with excessive alcohol intake is particularly treatable. As the Journal goes on to say: "In all types of dementia, adequate nutrition may improve physical well-being, help maximize the patient's functioning, and improve the quality of life."

Some studies indicate nutritional deficiencies may be a problem for almost 40% of the over 80 population. And, nearly half of all nursing home patients have been shown to have some vitamin or mineral deficiency. These lower than normal levels of vitamins and minerals are important because they contribute to loss of mental ability. For example, memory loss is more frequent in patients who have lower than normal blood levels of vitamin B-12 and folate.

Preserve memory with good nutrition;

Apple cider vinegar supplies a balanced dose of vital amino acids, vitamins, and minerals that both the mind and body need for good health.

One of the worst, and best known, of the mind robbing diseases associated with aging is Alzheimer's disease (AD). Some studies show AD sufferers are particularly short of calcium, thiamin and niacin. And low serum B-12 levels have been reported in up to 30% of elderly patients with this kind of dementia. Almost every patient in a recent study of nutrient deficiencies showed complete recovery when given B-12 therapy. Folate supplements also proved valuable.

Thiamin deficiency is another nutritional cause of chronic memory problems. If the diet is sufficiently short of this nutrient, nerve cell loss and hemorrhages in the brain can result. Experts continue to remind us: "...dietary modification may play an important role in the control of several ...diseases that may produce a dementia..."

The more we learn about good nutrition and the importance of getting an assortment of vitamins and minerals each day, the easier it is to understand old-time reliance on apple cider vinegar. One grandmother suggests this way to a healthy old age: "Stir a teaspoon of apple cider vinegar and a teaspoon of honey into a glass of water and drink it with your meal. Do this 3 times a day to remain bright and alert all your life."

Treating malnutrition with megadoses of vitamins is being tested, with mixed results. Sometimes it is difficult to get the balanced dose a particular individual may need. And, there is always the possibility of doing harm by giving too many vitamins, or of giving an overdose of minerals. Vitamin therapy can also be expensive. It is much better to prevent nutrient shortages by eating a balanced diet. And, for balancing the diet, it is hard to match the nutritional storehouse contained in a tablespoon of old-fashioned, naturally good, apple cider vinegar.

HEALING & INVIGORATING VINEGARS

Many cultures use plants to brighten the memory and sharpen the mind. Vinegar based tonics combine these time tested folk remedies with its own goodness. Scented vinegar can be used to soothe, invigorate or arouse the senses. Other vinegars are also associated with love. And still other vinegars are used to strengthen the immune system, kill germs and aid healing. Some ways that have been said, down through the ages, to enhance vinegar's natural goodness by using it in combination with healing plants follow:

Ginkgo leaves make an excellent addition to vinegar; it is famous for its ability to perk up a deteriorating memory. If fresh plant leaves are not available for pickling, add ginkgo extract to vinegar and flavor it with a few garlic cloves.

A potion made by soaking the dried roots and leaves of the forest trillium in apple cider vinegar has long been used to hasten the healing of leg ulcers. It is also said to ease the discomfort of varicose veins and hemorrhoids.

TCM = Traditional Chinese Medicine.

Traditional Chinese Medicine practitioners

recommend eating an umeboshi plum each day. These extremely tart and salty, pickled fruits are considered a morning wake-up tonic for the mind.

Add a large handful of red clover blossoms to a nice sized bottle of apple cider vinegar and allow to age for a couple of weeks. The resulting liquid will have an aroma capable of arousing the senses. Put a few drops into a glass of water to make a tonic that will give you a sense of well being while it strengthens the respiratory system and discourages coughs. This delightful brew is also healing to skin disorders such as psoriasis and eczema; simply pat it on to irritated skin areas and you will soon feel much better.

A healing elixir to pat onto rheumatic joints can be prepared by adding fresh young tomato leaves to vinegar. A very small amount of this vinegar, sprinkled over food, is said to calm digestive disorders.

Add several sprigs of lavender to warm vinegar and you will have a powerfully scented mixture that will encourage feelings of desire. Sprinkle a few drops on pillowcases to promote peaceful sleep.

For a vinegar that is reputed to stimulate feelings of love, slice a few pieces of licorice root into a bottle of apple cider vinegar and age for at least two weeks before using.

Make a strong garlic tonic to increase passion by filling a bottle with peeled garlic cloves, cover with vinegar and age. This potion was once considered so potent some religious orders banned it.

Onion flavored vinegar is both a culinary delight and an elixir long reputed to energize the libido. Use tiny whole onions or neatly sliced ones for an attractive bottle of goodness. If you use white or clear rice vinegar the onions will remain snowy white and appetizing.

Make a healing elixir to awaken warm and loving feelings by soaking the flowers and small twigs of the Chinese cinnamon in apple cider vinegar. A small dash of this added to a salad will also perk up the appetite and chase away the fevers of colds.

Boost confidence and feeling of well being with a sprinkling of vinegar enhanced with the blossoms of the pink monkey flower.

Scrapings from the dried roots of the vanilla scented heliotrope, sometimes called valerian, is one of nature's most well-known sleep aids. Use it to make a vinegar tonic that will induce relaxation and calmness and serve as a gentle aid to pleasant dreams.

Eastern medicine uses Gotu Kola leaves and their B vitamins to fight stress and to treat mentally handicapped children and unstable adults. It is also considered an aid for enhancing memory. It must work, after all, elephants eat it! The dried stems and leaves, added to apple cider vinegar, produce a healing potion said to promote faster healing of skin diseases and abrasions. This plant is sometimes known as Indian pennywort.

Low iron in the most common nutritional deficiency.

VINEGAR AND IRON

Children, adolescents and women of child bearing age should be sure to consume generous amounts of foods that are high in iron. The U.S. Surgeon General stresses that iron deficiency is a special problem for those in low-income families.

Others who should be sure they are getting lots of iron in their diets are high users of aspirin. Aspirin frequently causes intestinal blood loss, making the person at risk for iron deficiency.

One long-standing solution to low iron intake is to cook in iron pots. Each time one of these pans is used, some iron leaches into food. The higher the acid content of foods, the more iron will be absorbed into food. Adding a splash of vinegar to meats, sauces, and stews will raise their acid content and so increase the amount of iron they leach from iron pans.

To prevent anemia, the body needs iron, B-12, folate and a wide range of other nutrients. Apple cider vinegar delivers many of these nutrients, in an easy to digest and absorbable form.

The average adult diet includes only about 50% of the recommended level of calcium

VINEGAR AND CALCIUM

Calcium is the most abundant mineral in the human body. Besides its well-known part in forming bones, calcium is necessary for many other parts of the body to work properly. Although only 1% of the body's calcium is found outside the skeleton, without this small amount muscles do not contract properly, blood clotting is affected and neural function is seriously impaired.

Calcium absorption is affected by the amount of certain other substances in the body. For example, a diet too rich in phosphorus can cause calcium not to be absorbed properly. Or, eating too much protein can interfere with calcium absorption. Then, even if enough calcium is eaten, the body cannot draw it out of food and use it.

Each year over 300,000 women suffer fractured hips. 200,000 will never return to normal life. Nearly 45,000 will die within six months of the fractures from complications. Other thousands find their spinal column begins to collapse, reducing height and producing the back deformity known as a widow's hump. Osteoporosis is a major factor in these disabling fractures.

As the body ages it is less and less efficient at pulling calcium from food. Complicating this is the fact that with age, people tend to take in less and less calcium. Some of this is because many older individuals develop lactose intolerance, causing them to drop calcium-rich dairy products from their diets.

And so it comes as no surprise that many individuals find their bones begin to shrink as they get older. As osteoporosis advances, bones decrease in both size and density. The result is porous, fragile bones that fracture easily. It is a serious health problem, causing deformity, disability, and pain. Bones, you see, are living tissue. They are constantly being rebuilt and replaced. Whenever there is a shortage of calcium in muscles, blood, or nerves, the body pulls it from bones.

Apple cider vinegar contains a trace of needed calcium. It can also be used to dissolve calcium in soup bones. Several recent scientific reports show that when vinegar is added to the water in which soup bones are cooked, it leaches calcium from the bones and deposits it in the soup stock!

Some time-honored ways to combine vinegar and calcium, and some new ways medical research validates vinegar's use follow:

Calcium-Rich Chicken Soup
1/2   cup vinegar
2 to 3 lbs. chicken bones
1/2   cup minced onion
3/4   cup tiny pasta
  2   bouillon cubes
  2   slightly beaten egg whites
  2   tablespoons freshly chopped parsley
To make a delicious, low calorie, calcium-rich chicken soup, begin with a gallon of water and at least 1/2 cup vinegar. Gently simmer 2 or 3 pounds of bones (chicken wings are a good choice) for about 2 hours, uncovered. Strain the broth and skim off all fat. Strip the

meat from the bones and add the chicken, onion, pasta, and bouillon cubes to the stock. Bring to a boil and cook for 10 minutes. Remove from heat and immediately dribble the egg whites into the hot liquid, stirring continuously. Mix in the parsley and serve. This soup is low calorie, healthy and it adds calcium to the diet!

Calcium-Rich Vegetable Beef Soup
Beef bones
2 garlic cloves
Chopped onions
    Cover beef bones (the remains of a prime rib roast, a pound or two of short ribs or couple of knuckle bones work well) with a gallon of water with 1/2 cup of vinegar, a medium onion and 2 peeled garlic cloves added to it. Gently simmer for 2 or 3 hours, skim off all fat, strain the broth and return a cup or two of small pieces of beef to the pot. Add remaining ingredients and boil until all is tender. Remaining ingredients can be any combination of: fresh or dried parsley, basil, fresh or canned tomatoes, celery, cabbage, spinach, onion, corn, peas, green beans, carrots, potatoes, barley and salt if you must.

Research indicates cooking longer than 2 hours does not add much extra calcium

    As little as one tablespoon of vinegar per quart of water can make a difference in the amount of calcium that is pulled from boiled soup bones. A stronger vinegar solution (such as those used above) results in even more calcium being added to soup!

Calcium-Rich Salads
    Another way to add calcium to the diet is to crumble feta cheese over torn greens. Use spinach, collards, beet tops and kale, in addition to lettuce leaves. Sprinkle on a mixture of 2 tablespoons apple cider vinegar, 2 tablespoons honey, and 2 tablespoons water.

Caution: Those taking blood-thinning medicines need to limit their intake of dark green vegetables such as spinach and kale.

Calcium Supplements
    Newest research describes calcium supplements as being useful in the prevention and treatment of osteoporosis. And so, many doctors and nutritionists recommend them. Calcium supplements are prescribed for those with calcium deficient diets, elders who do not metabolize calcium adequately and for those with increased calcium needs (this can include postmenopausal

Osteoporosis is literally porus bones!

women). This calcium is usually added to the diet by taking calcium tablets or anti-acid tablets.

The US Pharmacopoeia Convention sets standards for drugs. It says an effective calcium tablet should dissolve in a maximum time of 30 minutes. An anti-acid tablet should be completely broken down in 10 minutes. If a tablet takes longer to break up than the recommended time, its usefulness is seriously impaired.

Studies estimate that more than half of the popular calcium supplements on the market do not meet this recommended timetable. Yet, the body can only properly use calcium supplements if they disintegrate in a reasonable length of time after being taken.

A simple to use vinegar test can tell you whether or not your calcium supplement dissolves in time for your body to digest it properly:

- Drop the calcium supplement tablet into three ounces of room temperature vinegar.
- Stir briskly, once every five minutes.
- At the end of 30 minutes the tablet should be completely disintegrated.

Tests by medical researchers found that times varied widely among the most popular brands. One brand of calcium supplement tablet broke up, completely, in three minutes. Another popular brand tablet was still mostly intact after 30 minutes.

15 to 20 million Americans suffer from osteoporosis.

OSTEOPOROSIS

About 20 million Americans are affected by osteoporosis. This contributes to the more than a million bone fractures, every year, that occur in individuals over 45 years old. Over the years, this adds up to a lot of disability. For example, one out of every three women over 65 has at least one fractured vertebra. When these tiny back bones crack, they can cause disabling pain.

Hip fractures are an even bigger problem. By 90 years of age, one out of every six men and one out of every three women will have suffered a fractured hip. One out of each five hip fractures leads to death. Long term nursing care is required for many others. All told, osteoporosis costs this country many billions of dollars every year.

As the body ages, the stomach produces less acid. Some believe this fact contributes to calcium shortages in elders. After all, acid is needed to dissolve almost all calcium supplement tablets. One solution may be to take calcium supplements with an old-fashioned vinegar tonic. It not only has acid for dissolving calcium, it adds the bit of extra that is in vinegar!

VINEGAR AND BORON

Have you had your boron today? If you began the day with apple cider vinegar your body is probably well fortified against boron deficiency. This critical trace element is needed for good health and strong bones.

Boron is a mineral that is necessary for both plant and animal life. When it is not readily available to plants, they do not grow properly. Some become dwarfs and others crack and become disfigured. The human body does not make strong, straight bones when it is missing from the diet. One reason for this is that boron plays a critical role in the way the body uses calcium. Without boron, calcium cannot form and maintain strong bones.

When vinegar releases its boron into the body, all sorts of wonderfully healthy things begin to happen. Boron affects the way steroid hormones are released. Then it regulates both their use and how long they stay active in the body.

How boron builds bones is just now beginning to be understood by scientists. One of the few things they do know is it makes changes in the way the membrane around individual cells works.

The boron and hormone connection is vital to bone formation. Blood and tissue levels of several steroid hormones (such as estrogen and testosterone) increase dramatically in the presence of boron. Both of these are needed to complete the calcium-to-bone growth cycle. This relationship between hormones, boron and calcium helps to explain why estrogen replacement is sometimes one of the treatments considered for battling osteoporosis.

Some other trace elements necessary for maintaining bone mass are manganese, silicon, and magnesium. Some doctors recommend supplements of all of them for post-menopausal women, even though no one knows exactly how they work. Many feel boron is useful for treating a lot of the ailments (such as arthritis) that doctors are not able to treat successfully with drugs.

One thing that we do know is that apple cider vinegar supplies boron, as well as manganese, silicon and magnesium to the body. Even more important, it does so in a balanced-by-nature way.

Herbal & Fortified Vinegars

Some scientists believe vinegar (acetic acid) was part of the primordial soup of life. It is present in most plant and animal tissues. Even the human body makes some, as it is needed to burn both fats and carbohydrates. It also plays a role in how the body stores fat. When vinegar enters the blood stream it is carried to the kidneys and muscles. There, it is either oxidized into pure energy or used to make body tissues, through its ability to help form essential amino acids.

VINEGAR IS PART OF A HEALTHY DIET!

Apple cider vinegar has been featured in folklore for centuries as an aid to good health. Today, thousands of devoted believers still take a daily tonic of apple cider vinegar. The traditional dose is one teaspoon of apple cider vinegar and one teaspoon of honey, stirred into a glass of water and taken twice a day. Another way to take vinegar is to stir a teaspoon each of vinegar and honey into a full quart of water and then use this as a substitute for expensive sports drinks.

IT'S NOT YOUR GRANDMOTHER'S VINEGAR

If you think of vinegar as merely the pucker in pickles or the zip in salad dressings you are in for a wonderful surprise. New vinegar-based taste sensations – called fortified vinegars – blend its bold taste with fruit and vegetable purees. The result is amazing! Fortified vinegars are thick and tangy, intensely flavored and packed with healthy vitamins, minerals and fiber. In addition to perking up salads, these new vinegars make great no fat, no cholesterol toppings for fruit, vegetable, fish and meat dishes.

Fortified vinegars offer a way to combine the tremendous nutritional benefits of fruits and vegetables with the goodness of vinegar. Whole fruits and vegetables are used, so all their vitamins, minerals, enzymes and the hundreds of other components are preserved. These nutrient packed vinegars taste good and add color and zest to unexciting foods. Try one of them today!

Try a nutrient packed fortified vinegar today.

Fortified vinegars begin with fruits and vegetables that are pureed in a blender, then the puree is combined with good, wholesome vinegar. The result is a mild, pleasantly colored dressing that tastes satisfying without the need for high calorie, artery clogging oils. These new vinegars offer a way to combine the tremendous nutritional benefits of fruits and vegetables with the healthy goodness of vinegar. Because whole fruits and vegetables are used, their vitamins, minerals, enzymes and phytocompounds are preserved. Fortified vinegars are so packed with fruit and vegetable goodness that when you use a generous portion of it on your food it can add an entire extra serving of fruit or vegetable to your meal. These taste delights are an easy way to get a daily dose of vinegar, perk up bland foods and – most of all – they are just plain good tasting!

Herbs and spices may be added, too. To prepare the recipes that follow, simply blend all ingredients until they are smooth and free of chunks. The intensity of flavor that is best for you may vary from that of others. So, some optional seasonings are listed. Feel free to experiment with these recipes to produce your own personal variations. They make great dips, dressings for salads or marinades.

A WORD ABOUT HEAT . . .
When using organic products that have not been pasteurized to make specialty vinegars, do not use heat, as it can harm nutrients. Heat can also deplete aromatics. When using supermarket varieties of apple cider vinegar, this care is not needed, as it has already been heated in the pasteurizing process.

PREPARING FORTIFIED VINEGARS

To prepare fortified vinegars, simply blend all ingredients in the recipes that follow until they are smooth and creamy. Usually, this requires putting them in a blender. They make great dips, dressings for salads, marinades and toppings for other foods. Experiment with these recipes to produce your own personal variations. The intensity of flavor that is best for you may vary from that of others, so some optional seasonings are listed.

Specialty vinegars can be thick and creamy or clear and sparkling. They can look like ordinary vinegar, or be brightened with leafy sprigs and chunks of colorful food. Thick, dense mixtures are usually called fortified and clear ones are called herbal. The ingredients for making some of the most wholesome of fruit and vegetable vinegars, the fortified ones, follow:

Fortified Honey-Apple Vinegar Tonic
2   Medium apples
1/2   Cup apple cider vinegar
1/4   Cup honey
      If you take a daily tonic of apple cider vinegar and honey, a tablespoon of this dressing is an especially appetizing way to do it. For maximum nutritional benefits use immediately. Optional ingredients: 1/2 teaspoon cinnamon; 1/4 teaspoon nutmeg; an additional 1/4 cup honey. In addition to all the health inducing goodness of apple cider vinegar and honey this combination adds the nutritional benefits of fresh apples. Included in the nearly 400 substances that have been identified in apples are: calcium, beta carotene, carotenoids, chlorophyll, fiber, folacin, fructose, glucose, clycine, lecithin, lysine, pectin, niacin, selenium, sorbitol, sucrose, thiamin, tryptophan and zinc.

Cucumber-Celery

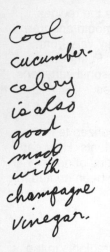

Cool cucumber-celery is also good made with champagne vinegar.

1   Large cucumber
2   Cups celery
1   Cup rice vinegar
1   Cup water
      Good for seasoning steamed vegetables, boiled potatoes or pasta. Optional ingredient: 1/2 teaspoon salt. In addition to all the nutrients in vinegar this combination adds the goodness of fresh cucumbers and celery. Included in the nearly 450 substances that have been identified in celery and the more than 175 substances that have been identified in cucumbers are: calcium, beta carotene, carotenes, choline, copper, coumarin, beta-elemene, glycine, histidine, iron, lysine, riboflavin, tryptophan, tyrosine, beta amyrin, fluorine, folacin, selenium, beta-sitosterol and thiamin.

Garlic
8   Garlic bulbs
1   Cup apple cider vinegar
      Bake fresh, whole garlic bulbs until tender. Peel away the outer skin and squeeze the soft garlic paste into a blender. Blend in the

apple cider vinegar. Optional ingredients: 1/2 to 1 cup oil, 1/2 to 1 teaspoon salt, 2 teaspoons sugar, 2 teaspoons dry mustard. In addition to all the nutrients in vinegar this combination adds the goodness of fresh garlic. Included in the more than 275 substances that have been identified in garlic are: ascorbic acid, calcium, beta carotene, copper, fiber, clycine, lysine, niacin, riboflavin, selenium and thiamin.

Raspberry
1   Cup raspberries
3   Tablespoons red wine vinegar
    Raspberries may be fresh or frozen, sweetened or unsweetened. Great over ice cream, peaches, melon slices or fruit salad. Make a vinegar sundae by spooning it over ice cream, or use it as a topping of pancakes. Make an old-fashioned Raspberry Sipper by stirring one tablespoon fortified raspberry vinegar into a tall glass of cold water. Drink this delicious liquid one-half hour before mealtime. You will add a bit of vinegar to your diet and the pre-meal drink will help control your appetite. In addition, it really tastes good! In addition to all the nutrients in vinegar this combination adds the goodness of red raspberries. Included in the more than 100 substances that have been identified in red raspberries are: acetic acid, ascorbic acid, boron, calcium, beta carotene, chromium, fiber, lactic acid, pectin, riboflavin, salicylic acid, selenium, tannin and thiamin.

Cucumber-Onion
  1   Large cucumber
1/2   Cup red wine vinegar
1/4   Cup onion
    No need to peel a well-scrubbed cucumber or remove the seeds. Optional ingredients: 1/4 to 1/2 cup oil or replace the red wine with champagne vinegar. In addition to all the nutrients in vinegar and cucumbers, this recipe adds the goodness of onions. Included in the nearly 350 substances that have been identified in onions are: ascorbic acid, calcium, beta carotene, choline, fiber, lysine, niacin, pectin, riboflavin, selenium and sulfur.

Cucumber, Celery & Onion Vinegar
1   Large cucumber
2   Cups celery
1   Small onion
1   Cup champagne Vinegar
1   Cup water
Optional Ingredient: 1/2 Teaspoon Salt.
    Serve this drizzled generously over chunks of fresh tomatoes. It is good for seasoning steamed vegetables, boiled potatoes or pasta,

too. To make Cucumber Boats, cut cucumbers lengthwise and scoop out their seeds. Fill with a mixture made of equal parts of this fortified vinegar, yogurt, diced tomatoes and celery.

Strawberry
1   Cup strawberries
1/4   Cup champagne vinegar
  This is a mildly tart vinegar that is high in vitamin C. Optional ingredients are 1/2 cup yogurt or 2 tablespoons honey.

Carrot

Cooking carrots increases their beta carotene!

  1 Cup carrots
1/2 Cup apple cider vinegar
1/2 Cup water
3 to 4 Tablespoons honey (optional)
  Use raw carrots for a cool vegetable dip, cooked ones for a smoother sauce to top cooked foods or add to soups. In addition to all the nutrients in vinegar this recipe adds the goodness of carrots. Included in the more than 400 substances that have been identified in carrots are: ascorbic acid, boron, calcium, citric acid, copper, glycine, lecithin, lysine, niacin, riboflavin, selenium, thiamin, tryptophan, vitamin B-6, vitamin D and vitamin E. Plus, carrots contain alpha, beta, epsilon and gamma carotenes.

Honeydew
2   Cups honeydew melon
1/4   Cup champagne vinegar
1/4   Cup water
  This is an excellent topping for fruits and ices. Optional ingredients: 1 tablespoon honey or 1/4 teaspoon ginger.

Lemon
1   Lemon
2   Tablespoons champagne vinegar
1/2   Cup water
  Use the entire lemon, both pulp and peeling. Excellent splashed on sea food. Optional ingredient: 1 cup cabbage.

Parsley
2   Cups fresh parsley
1/2   Cup red wine vinegar
1/2   Cup water
  This bright green vinegar goes well with meats and steamed vegetables.

Kale-Mustard

2 Cups kale, fresh or cooked
1/4 Cup apple cider vinegar
1/4 Cup water
2 Tablespoons dry mustard
This is a thick and healthy dip or a topping for vegetables.
Optional ingredient: 15 peppercorns.

Mint Sauce

2 Cups fresh mint leaves
1 Cup apple cider vinegar
2 Tablespoons honey
Malt or red wine vinegar may be substituted.

Golden Peach

Cook 2 cups peeled, chopped peaches in 1 cup water and 1 cup sugar. When the peaches are tender add 2 teaspoons vanilla, mix well in a blender and stir into 1 cup vinegar. Especially good diluted and served as a cold soup!

Thick Strawberry

Combine in a blender, 2 cups fresh strawberries, 1 cup sugar and 1/2 cup vinegar. Mix well and serve with fruit or sliced cold meats.

HERB & SPICE VINEGARS

Herbal vinegars are tasty ways to add healing, healthful nutrients to meals. Make your own from standard apple cider, rice, wine or champagne vinegar and save on the high cost of these specialty vinegars! Some ways to make some of the best — and most popular — herb and spice vinegars follow:

Sparkling Garlic

Peel two cloves fresh garlic and add to 1 quart apple cider vinegar. Allow to set for 6 weeks before using. Add more garlic for a stronger vinegar.

Quickest Herbal Vinegar

Heat a quart of apple cider vinegar in a glass pan until it is almost ready to boil. Put an herbal tea bag in a bottle, pour the hot vinegar into the bottle and cap. When cool, remove the tea bag. The vinegar is ready to use immediately.

Rich Blueberry

Add 2 cups blueberries to 1 cup boiling water. Simmer until the fruit is tender. Add 1 1/2 cup sugar and stir until crystals are dissolved. Strain and add to 1 quart vinegar along with 1 teaspoon allspice and a few fresh, whole berries.

Green Onion

Trim the roots and 1 inch off the top of 3 small green onions. Push them into a quart of vinegar and replace the cap. Let set for 3 weeks and then remove the onions. For stronger taste, repeat the process with new onions

Hot! Hot! Pepper

Wash and prick a dozen small cayenne peppers. Add to a quart of red wine vinegar and allow to set for a month before using. As the vinegar is used, it can be replaced with fresh vinegar.

Sweet Pepper

Place 1 cup each sweet red and green bell peppers, cut in 1/2 inch strips, in a quart bottle. Cover with vinegar and age for 3 weeks before using.

Pretty Parsley

Stuff several large sprigs of parsley into a pint of champagne vinegar and age for 4 weeks before using.

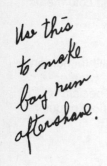
Use this to make bay rum aftershave.

Crystal Clear Parsley

Heat 1 pint of rice vinegar to the boiling point and pour over 1/2 cup dried parsley. Allow to steep for 2 weeks, then strain through a cloth.

Garlic & Chili

Chop 4 garlic cloves into a bottle. Add 2 tablespoons chili powder and 1/2 teaspoon each of paprika, cumin and cloves. Fill the bottle with vinegar and set aside for 3 weeks. Strain and use sparingly.

Dramatic Dill

Add 3 large heads of dill to a quart of vinegar. Will be ready to use in about 3 weeks.

Onion & Curry

Add 1 sliced onion and 3 tablespoons curry powder to a pint of vinegar and set aside for 4 weeks. Strain through a cloth before using.

Fresh Mint

Pack a pint bottle with freshly bruised mint leaves. Cover with vinegar and age for 3 weeks before using.

Tangy Tarragon

Add 2 sprigs of fresh tarragon to a pint of mild rice vinegar. After 3 weeks replace the tarragon with 1 fresh spring and use immediately.

Anise

This relative of fennel has a sweet, licorice-like taste and pretty fernlike leaves. Add few sprigs to rice vinegar and it will be ready to use in two weeks.

Bay

Leaves of the sweet bay tree are shiny and dark green. Their flavor goes well with meats. For an extra strong seasoning vinegar, pack fresh or dried bay leaves in a jar and cover with vinegar. Begin using in 1 week.

Ginger

Even in very small amounts, ginger adds a lot of flavor. Use this unusual tasting condiment in Oriental dishes. A small piece will flavor a pint of vinegar.

Horseradish

A few slivers of horseradish root in a pint of vinegar will produce an especially zippy flavored brew in a week or two. Add extra horseradish for a zestier result.

Sweet Marjoram

This Old World herb is very strong and makes a vinegar that can pep up a bland stew or soup. Add a handful of leaves to a pint of apple cider vinegar and age for at least 2 weeks.

Exotic Ginger

Place 1/2 cup chopped ginger in a pint of vinegar and set aside for 4 weeks. Strain, then add a small piece of ginger to the bottle. Use immediately.

Spicy Nasturtium

Add 1 packed cup of bruised nasturtium leaves and flowers to a quart of white wine vinegar. After 3 weeks, strain and add a dozen fresh flowers before using.

Sleepy Lavender

Put 6 sprigs of lavender in a quart bottle and cover with clear vinegar. After 6 weeks it will be ready to use. A mist of this on a pillow is said to induce sound sleep.

Golden Marigold

Fill a quart bottle with fully opened marigolds and cover with clear vinegar. Let set for 4 weeks and strain. Add 5 or 6 fresh flowers to the bottle and use this strong infusion as a scented spray.

Other herbs for making vinegars are dill, basil, rosemary, mint, catnip, lemon balm, sage, tarragon, caraway and thyme. Combine several herbs to create your own special flavors. Then add a dash of cloves, allspice, nutmeg or cinnamon.

CAUTION! Many foods and flowers are sprayed with dangerous insecticides and will need to be thoroughly washed.

HEALING HERBAL VINEGARS

Those of the ancient world quickly learned to combine vinegar with beneficial plants for maximum medicinal value. Herb vinegars have been in use for thousands of years. Yet, the virtues of healing herbs are only now beginning to be understood by the scientific community. Herbal vinegars can be prepared easily by simply adding fresh or dried herbs to white, wine or apple cider vinegar. Let the herbs steep in the vinegar for 2 to 4 weeks before using. Herbs may be strained out, or left in.

Dandelion adds its mild laxative nature to vinegar's natural antiseptic qualities. It also has an anti-inflammatory effect on the intestines. This is an old time remedy for ailments of the pancreas and liver, said to ease jaundice and cirrhosis. It is also a diuretic, and as such is considered useful in lowering blood pressure. (Dandelion is rich in potassium, a mineral some other diuretics pull out of the body.)

Myrrh has long been considered of particular value in maintaining a healthy mouth. Swish this vinegar around in the mouth to hasten healing of sores and to soothe red, swollen gums. This will also sweeten the breath. Ancients used it for treating chest congestion.

Sage vinegar not only adds its delicate hint of flavoring to meats, it tenderizes them. Splashed into soups and dressings, it serves up a tranquilizer for frazzled nerves.

Peppermint, like all the mints, settles and calms the digestive system. Use a couple of teaspoons of peppermint vinegar, added to a glass of water, to ease stomach cramps, diarrhea, or gas. Add a teaspoon of honey and it is one of the best tasting cures for indigestion. Mix this herb vinegar with others to intensify their flavor and effectiveness.

Rosemary, the herb of remembrance, combines with healthy, amino acid laced apple cider vinegar to treat maladies of the head. It boosts the function of mind and memory, relieves tension headaches, and eases dizziness.

Eucalyptus is the source of the eucalyptol, which makes some cough drops so effective. Steam from vinegar that has absorbed the aromatic oil of this herb helps to clear a stuffy head or a clogged respiratory system. A popular over-the-counter salve for relieving the stiffness and swelling of arthritis and rheumatism carries the distinctive aroma of eucalyptus.

Wormwood is quite bitter. This vinegar is best used externally, as a deterrent to fleas and other insects, or applied as a wound dressing. For insect control, sprinkle it liberally onto infested areas of rooms.

Rue was once given as an antidote for poison mushrooms and toadstools, as well as the bite of snakes, spiders, and bees. Bitter, aromatic rue vinegar was once sprinkled about to ward off both witches and contagious diseases.

Lavender makes a vinegar that is pleasantly aromatic and useful for fighting off anxiety attacks. The haunting scent of lavender as long been associated with headache relief and calming of stressed nerves.

Thyme vinegar is a good addition to meat dishes, as it both flavors and tenderizes. Applied to the body, it acts to deter fungus growth.

Spearmint is one of the gentler mints. A bit of spearmint vinegar in a glass of water calms the stomach and digestive system. It also relieves gas and adds a tangy zing to iced tea.

Clove vinegar is especially good for stopping vomiting. Its use dates back more than 2,000 years (to China) where it was considered an aphrodisiac.

Cloves are the dried buds of the clove tree.

When herb vinegars are used for medicinal purposes, the usual dose is one to three teaspoons added to a full glass of water. They can also be sprinkled into meat and vegetable dishes or splashed on salads. The very strong vinegars, and the very bitter ones, should be used sparingly, and only for eternal purposes.

WHY TO USE HERBAL VINEGARS

When you enliven the taste of food with herbal vinegars, you add more than flavor. Many herbs are believed to have healing qualities. Some of the best known of the healing herbs follow:

Garlic activates the natural killer cells of the immune system. It also helps to preserve eye function and detoxify pollutants such as lead.

Parsley contains the flavonoid, apigenin, a free radical scavenger.

Purple Coneflower (echinacea) boosts immune system response by improving white blood cell count. It is credited with being able to rouse the body's defenses when threatened by flu symptoms.

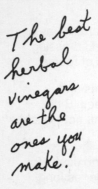
The best herbal vinegars are the ones you make!

Purslane is the best plant source of the immune system building Omega 3 acids for which fish oils are known. It is also credited with contributing to the healthy gums needed to retain teeth in old age.

Lemon vinegar goes well with many foods and has strong antioxidant properties!

Some other healthy reasons to add fortified vinegars to the diet follow:

Researchers in Finland say a diet enhanced with a wide variety of vitamins reduces the side effects of both radiation therapy and chemotherapy.

Lung cancer recovery rates are better for those who supplement their diets with vitamins such as those found in fortified vinegars. These include vitamins A, B-6, B-12, C, E and D, beta-carotene, thiamin, riboflavin, niacinamide, calcium, manganese, magnesium, zinc, copper, selenium, chromium and potassium.

Adding vitamin C to the diet can lower the body's production of allergy producing histamine by as much as one third.

Resistance to all kinds of infection is greater when the diet contains a wide variety of vitamins.

Normal amounts of zinc, such as the kind found in apple cider vinegar, are needed to keep the body feeling truly vigorous and full of life in old age. It is also important to maintaining fertility.

Eating lots of cauliflower fortified vinegar will give the body extra amounts of biotin. This plant-based nutrient helps it grow strong nails.

In A Pickle
And Proud Of It!

*I*t's the law: if the label says pickled, then the product must be put up in vinegar!

Our world would be very different without vinegar's lively flavor to perk up humdrum foods. Each year, Americans use hundreds of millions of gallons of vinegar. It is used alone, in pickling, and in innumerable condiments. Almost half of U.S. households buy some vinegar each year mostly in the summertime. The pint size bottle is the most popular, followed by the quart size. Twice as much white vinegar as apple cider vinegar is sold. The retail market accounts for only about a third of vinegar's total sales; the remainder in used to make other products, such as pickles, mustard and catsup.

The best vinegars begin with healthful, natural foods and the Food and Drug Administration (FDA) says it has to have at least a 4% acetic acid content. And, the government treats different grades of vinegar differently. For example, there are differences in the way taxes and import duties are levied. Quality vinegar, from expensive food based sources such as fruit juices, honey, maple syrup, apples, grapes or even sugar cane or corn are subject to a higher tax rate than lower quality vinegars. Different tax treatment dates way back in time. In England, the Revenue Acts established during the reign of Charles II charged different duties on beer and on vinegar-beer.

Charles II reigned in the 1600's.

Besides the differences in nutritional values, grain and spirit vinegars do not compare in taste to good, high-quality vinegars. A quality vinegar has a sour taste, without being bitter. Sour tastes are one of the sensations the body is most able to detect. The sensitive sides of the tongue (the area where sour is registered) can detect one sour part in 130,000. But it is even more sensitive to bitter flavors. The tongue can detect one bitter part out of 2 billion. This sensitivity is a safety measure, to alert the body to poisons. It also makes cheap vinegars unpleasant to the tongue.

Good, sour, acidy vinegar causes saliva to flow. This increases the ability to taste and enjoy other foods. It also aids digestion.

Pickling, for example, is one of the most basic and easiest ways to preserve edibles. It works by increasing foods' acidity. Expect a batch of pickled vegetables to last a month or two in the refrigerator or over a year if they are canned. Because pickles are already partially preserved, they do not have to be canned in a pressure cooker. A boiling water bath provides enough heat to seal and sterilize them. Care does need to be taken in choosing containers. The high acid content reacts with some metals, such as aluminum and iron. It is better to use enamel, glass or stainless steel pans.

Even the water which is combined with the vinegar can affect the quality of the pickled food. Water high in iron or sulfur will darken foods. Be sure food to be preserved is of high quality, not bruised or over ripe.

Pickling changed the way mankind ate for all time because vinegar inhibits the growth of microorganisms that cause food to spoil. Some of this is due to its acid, which prevents microbial growth. And, lactic and other organic acids are produced by friendly bacteria present on fruits and vegetables. These newly formed chemicals improve flavor, too. Vinegar also has nonacid preserving qualities, as do salt, sugar and spices, which are added to vinegar to boost its ability to preserve.

PERSONALIZING TASTE

Everyone has their own idea of what the perfect pickle should taste like. There are several things you can do to adjust the taste: vary the kind of vinegar used, add or delete sugar or change the spices. There are some things you do not want to do in your quest for preserving the perfect pickle. Do not combat vinegar's tartness by diluting the vinegar excessively. This will lower the acid content of the mixture and could result in spoiled pickles.

It is better to mask tartness by adding extra sugar. Since sugar helps to preserve the food, doing this will not create a risk of spoilage. Use brown sugar and the entire batch will change to a darker color. Use honey and the flavor will be heavy and rich.

The salt used for pickling should always be 'pickling salt' or 'kosher salt.' They are both free of the iodine and starch often found in table salt. Iodine in the salt will darken the pickles, and the starchy anti-caking additives in table salt will cause the liquid to be cloudy.

Make simple cucumber pickles or be creative and preserve eggplant, cauliflower, carrots, beans, onions, okra, Brussels sprouts, squash, beets, or asparagus. Even fruits can be pickled. Flavor your mix with oregano, bay, red pepper, turmeric, mustard seeds or dry mustard, garlic, basil, dill, peppercorns, bell peppers, hot peppers, onions or garlic.

You can pickle a peck of hot peppers in a flash.

Basic Pickling

Always use firm, young veggies, because they make the crunchiest pickled food. And never store cucumbers for pickling in the refrigerator because they deteriorate if stored below 50°. For the best tasting pickles cut off the blossom ends (opposite end from the stem) of cucumbers. There are concentrated enzymes in the flowering end of the cucumber and they can soften pickles. And, never boil vinegar for pickles any longer than absolutely necessary. Acetic acid evaporates at boiling temperatures, leaving a vinegar which is too weak to do a good job of preserving.

Try some of the following vinegary taste sensations and then perhaps you will want to develop some recipes of your own.

Sliced Cucumber Pickles

Slice lots of cucumbers and a few onions. Arrange them in a crock, in layers. Sprinkle salt over each layer. Add very cold water and let them set and become very crisp. While the cucumbers and onions soak, mix sugar, vinegar, and spices in an enamel pan. Bring the liquid to a boil and immediately remove from the heat. Drain the brine off the cucumbers and onions. Add the pickles to the hot spiced vinegar. Put the mixture into clean jars and boil. When cool, set the jars away for a few weeks before beginning to use the pickles. And remember, pickles pick up the flavor of whatever they are marinated in. This is what gives them their flavor.

Puckery Pickles

For truly tart and sour pickles, give them an extra helping of vinegar. Begin with a jar of whole dill pickles. Drain off the pickling juice and discard it. Next, cut the pickles into thin slices and put them back into the jar. Fill the jar with white vinegar and refrigerate for 5 days before eating. Pure puckery pleasure!

Tasty Pimientos

Pimientos are merely pickled sweet peppers! Make your own by thinly slicing sweet red peppers, blanching them to soften, and soaking in vinegar.

3/4 cup vinegar	dash of salt
3/4 cup water	4 garlic cloves
1/4 cup sugar	2 red peppers
1 teaspoon olive oil	

Simmer everything for the pimientos except the garlic and peppers for 10 minutes. Put the garlic and thinly sliced peppers into a glass jar, pour the hot liquid over them and marinate for 3 weeks. Enjoy! For an interesting change, use green peppers, or mix red and green half and half for a bright holiday look.

Chutney

Chutney is made by combining chopped vegetables, fruits and spices in a sweet pickling liquid. Originally, it came from India, where it was made with mangoes, raisins, tamarinds, ginger, spices. In the United States and England it is more likely to be made with tomatoes, apples, gooseberries, peaches, or bananas. Serve chutneys with cold meats.

Traditionally, pickled foods are served at the beginning of a meal because they stimulate the flow of saliva and gastric juices. This makes other foods taste better. Exact amounts of spices, salt, sugar, and vinegar will depend on your own judgment. What tastes great to one person will be too tart, or too sweet, or too garlicky to another. Do not be afraid to experiment. Pickled foods are sturdy, able to withstand a lot of variation in the way they are processed. However, occasionally things do go wrong. The finished product is not perfect. Too strong or too weak a vinegar solution, or the wrong balance of sugar or salt can result in pickles that are not crisp and crunchy. Contact with minerals can cause pickles to turn unusual colors. Use the following information to identify the cause of pickling problems.

WHAT CAN GO WRONG?

If:	Pickles will be:
Pickling solution is too strong	Tough
Brine is too weak	Soft
Table salt is used	Cloudy
Pickling solution is too strong	Shriveled
Too much sugar	Shriveled
Too much salt	Tough ·
Cucumbers are old	Hollow
Cooked in a copper kettle	Off Color
Insufficient time in brine solution	Slippery
Water has a high mineral content	Off color
Cooked too long	Mushy

Vinegar can be fun! A Louisiana firm now produces some very special pickles. Called Upside-Down Cajun Brand Pickles, they come in rather ordinary looking glass jars. But, the labels are applied upside-down. This means, when the label is right-side-up, the lid is at the bottom. Supposedly, keeping pickle jars up-side-down keeps the pickles fresher!

The Vinegar Diet

*I*n recent times there has been an explosion of medical information. New ways of treating disease with drugs has driven food-based treatments into obscurity. The result, over the years, has been that much time-proven wisdom has been lost, forgotten or pushed aside. The notion that a well balanced diet was necessary for good health, as well as for weight control, was lost. And so *THE VINEGAR DIET* came into being! It is built around the fact that conventional 'dieting' is not the best way to regulate weight and health.

Diet *vs.* Dieting: Dieting can be a dangerous health concept. It has come to mean a special, temporary way of relating to food that somehow turns a flabby, prematurely aged, malnourished body into a slim, trim, youthful one. This is both untrue and unfortunate!

Untrue: Because it suggests a temporary change in eating can correct a lifetime of poor habits.

Unfortunate: Because it leads to impossible expectations and almost ensures failure. Throughout this volume the word 'diet' means a lifelong way of nourishing a healthy body, not a temporary attempt to alter weight. Changes in body mass which come about by following the guidelines of *THE VINEGAR DIET* should be lasting and health promoting. It is a realistic way to look better, feel better, be better!

VINEGAR IS PART OF A HEALTHY DIET!

Often vinegar is combined with honey in a tonic that

brings together the exceptional nutritional qualities of these two very special foods. Millions learned of this age-old tonic when its virtues were chronicled by physician D. C. Jarvis of Vermont. In Dr. Jarvis' book, FOLK MEDICINE, he praised the virtues of taking a daily tonic of apple cider vinegar and honey. His strong belief in the ability of apple cider vinegar to maintain an acid balance in the body was a large part of his faith in the tonic. His book stressed the common sense approach to food the Vermont country folk of his generation practiced. His "prescription" for maintaining health was to take, at least once a day:

2 Teaspoons apple cider vinegar
2 Teaspoons honey
Full glass of water

For those suffering from the pain of arthritis, rheumatism and other degenerative diseases he suggested the vinegar and honey combination be taken two to three times a day, with or before meals. Many people find a milder dose more palatable: 1 Teaspoon apple cider vinegar, 1 Teaspoon honey and Full glass of water

DO YOU NEED THE VINEGAR DIET?

Does your present diet supply everything you need for optimum health? Ask yourself:
- Are you as healthy as you want to be?
- Are you as healthy as you ought be?
- Are you as healthy as you can be?

Most Diets Are Nutritionally Inadequate!

Most likely, your diet does not supply enough of the nutrients needed for optimum health. It is estimated that less than 10% of the population follows the U.S. Agriculture Department's dietary guidelines. This means many do not get the Recommended Dietary Allowance (RDA) of important vitamins and minerals. And remember, the RDA gives only dietary minimums, the very smallest amount needed to prevent major diseases known to be caused by nutrient shortages. These amounts are not usually enough for maximum health. Studies show more than half of those admitted to a hospital have a nutritional deficiency.

Mature adults are particularly at risk for nutritional deficiencies because, as the body ages, it does not process foods as efficiently as it once did. And, the elderly tend to take more nutrient-depleting medications. To extend the good years as long as possible it is necessary to fight the effects of

RDA= is not always the optimum amount.

83

degenerative diseases. Extra amounts of many nutrients can increase vitality and vigor and retard some of the most obvious effects of aging. This can only be done by getting much more than the RDA of vitamins and minerals. The most frequently found nutrient shortages include: calcium, magnesium, thiamine, chromium, niacin, vitamin A, copper, potassium, vitamin B-12, folic acid, riboflavin, vitamins C & D, iron, selenium and zinc.

DEFICIENCY SYMPTOMS

CALCIUM deficiency has been linked to depression and loss of bone mass. Foods high in phosphorus, such as meat and carbonated drinks, increase the loss of calcium, as do salt and caffeine.

CHROMIUM shortfall can increase the risk of developing clogged arteries.

COPPER insufficiency increases the likelihood of getting infections and some arthritis has been linked to unusual copper levels.

FOLIC ACID deficiency increases with age and can cause fatigue and increased susceptibility to infection.

IRON deficiency is the most frequent cause of anemia and is associated with depression. It has even been linked to increased numbers of cold sores. As many as 80% of senior citizens have at least marginally low levels of iron.

MAGNESIUM shortfall can cause diminished heart function and can be part of the cycle involved in angina pain.

NIACIN insufficiency is particularly common among the elderly, especially those in institutions.

POTASSIUM deficit is associated with depression, muscle weakness and fatigue.

RIBOFLAVIN insufficiency is associated with depression and increased susceptibility to infection, perhaps because it is needed to metabolize protein.

SELENIUM shortfall little has been linked to an increased risk of cancer and clogged arteries.

THIAMINE insufficiency can cause slow healing of cuts and scrapes and can be a factor in depression.

Vitamin D helps bones absorb calcium.

VITAMIN A shortfall can lead to more frequent infections.

VITAMIN B-12 shortages of are linked to depression and excessive tiredness.

VITAMIN C deficiency is associated with depression, tiredness and insufficient synthesis of collagen (which may encourage the advance of arthritis). It is estimated that 40% of the women in the United States do not get enough of this nutrient.

VITAMIN D shortage of has been linked to bone

loss and can result in arthritis doing damage to cartilage at a faster rate than it would otherwise.

ZINC insufficiency can result in slow healing of cuts and scrapes and susceptibility to infection.

OVER SUPPLEMENTATION SYMPTOMS

Taking mega-doses of vitamins and minerals do not usually head off or cure health problems. Good nutrition is not that simple, because supplements can be risky. For example, everyone knows about the discomfort associated with too much acid in the stomach. But those with too little stomach acid are more susceptible to infections and parasites and are unable to properly absorb minerals such as calcium and iron. Only the proper balance aids digestion. Individual metabolism determines the amount of a nutrient that can cause dangerous side effects. Incorrectly used, the way a body processes food can change a supplemental nutrient into a possibly life-threatening poison. Nutrients also need to be taken in proper proportion to each other because they interact in ways that are not yet fully understood. Researchers do know that vitamins and minerals can be dangerous if taken improperly. Too much:

CALCIUM can interfere with the body's supply of vitamin K or its absorption of zinc.

COPPER can make the body more likely to get infections and lower the level of zinc.

FOLIC ACID compromises the availability of vitamin B-12 and zinc.

IRON can result in liver damage, nausea and lowered levels of zinc and vitamin E.

MAGNESIUM is associated with depression.

NIACIN can cause flushing and itching.

POTASSIUM can block the absorption of vitamin B-12.

SELENIUM can cause diarrhea, hair loss, easily broken fingernails and garlicky smelling breath; over supplementing can be fatal. It is hard to judge the amount of selenium in the diet because the natural content in food varies widely, depending on the soil where it was grown.

THIAMINE can result in itching and shortness of breath.

VITAMIN A increases feelings of fatigue, the risk of getting infections, headaches, brittle nails and causes yellow tinted skin.

VITAMIN B-12 can cause itching and interfere with vitamin B-6 absorption.

VITAMIN C can cause diarrhea.

Use fortified vinegars to get extra nutrients.

VITAMIN D can result in reduced kidney function as well as calcium deposits in joints and lungs.

ZINC can dampen the immune response and clock copper absorption.

CAUTION: If you are taking mega-doses of nutrients — do not suddenly stop taking them. A body that has adjusted itself to a high level of a particular vitamin or mineral may react to an abrupt change by developing deficiency symptoms. ALWAYS consult with a medical professional before making changes to your normal routine!

Popping Pills Is Not The Answer

A good diet provides a generous supply of all the substances the body needs to maintain health and fight disease. There can be hundreds of important nutrients in a single serving of wholesome food. A good diet will also go a long way toward keeping weight within normal limits. Getting balanced nutrients from food is what the vinegar diet is about! It is a lifelong system of eating — a way of living —and a philosophy of health! Its principles can be the beginning of a new tomorrow of personal health for you.

VINEGAR MAGIC

Good food contains more than the popular vitamins and minerals listed in most nutrient charts. In depth analysis of an ordinary apple reveals it contains more than 400 different substances! A single stalk of celery has nearly 450 identifiable components! Doctors do not yet know how the many substances in food work together in the body. They do know, when the body does not get everything it needs the result is sickness and wasting away of both tissue and bone. Even a marginal deficiency of a trace element or an essential nutrient can result in the body being unable to rebuild tissue and maintain the immune system.

The Magic Of Vinegar & Honey

Since the most ancient of times people believed certain foods can have dramatic — even supernatural or miraculous — effects on health and well being. Vinegar and honey have been among these marvels, perhaps because they supply so many different nutrients. A good, naturally produced apple cider vinegar contains far more than acetic acid. As apple juice ferments it produces a liquid laced with newly created alcohols, phenols and enzymes, while retaining tiny particles of apples with their storehouse of vitamins and minerals. Vinegar's enzymes are made by living bacteria. These enzymes are catalysts for biological reactions that are critical to life. The final result, that wonderful thing we call vinegar, has the goodness of the original food, plus much more! Often, the concentrated flower power of clover honey is included in vinegar tonics. This rich sweetness is an ideal companion to vinegar's puckery tartness. Honey is nature's original sweetener, containing an assortment of dissolved sugars such as sucrose, glucose and fructose. It also contains nearly 200 other substances, including minerals, vitamins, pigments, enzymes and amino acids.

Together, apple cider vinegar and honey provide a unique combination of health-promoting nutrients. Biochemists have now identified and measured hundreds of substances in the foods we eat, many of them minute amounts of trace elements. For a long time trace elements were ignored by most doctors and their importance to good health was underestimated. (Most nutrient charts list only the most plentiful and the most well known ones.)

Taking nutritional supplements is not the same as eating whole foods. The complex mix of phytochemicals in plants can not be duplicated chemically. And so, multivitamin and mineral pills include only a very few of the substances known to be necessary for life. If too much of some vitamins or minerals are taken it can be stored in the body and end up as a poison. Extra nutrients that are not stored in the body must be filtered out by the kidneys, causing them to work harder than they otherwise would have to. The safest way to get the goodness of food is through healthy eating habits.

CAN THE VINEGAR DIET BRING NEW HEALTH TO YOUR LIFE? VERY PROBABLY!

Eating better with the vinegar diet is about a whole lot more than vinegar! It is a complete way of living and feeling better about yourself! Best of all, you can begin today. Never again count calories, weigh food or struggle with measuring cups. The vinegar diet is as easy as filling your plate, as pleasant as eating your favorite food and as good for you as sunshine in the morning! *THE VINEGAR DIET* combines what we have always instinctively known about eating with the best of biochemical research. It is good food for a healthy body without:

Healthy goal = 30% (or less) calories from fat.

- Confusing calorie counting
- Complicated rules
- Depressing restrictions
- Fad foods
- Expensive supplements

Fifty years ago your Grandmother said, "Eat your fruits and vegetables." Twenty-five years ago your Mother said, "Eat your fruits and vegetables." Today's best scientific research confirms their wisdom. The very best health only comes when you – eat your fruits and vegetables!

Fruits and vegetables are the heart of healthy eating. And, many believe a daily vinegar tonic is also a good idea! Vinegar is an essential building block for the body. It can also help the body absorb the calcium it needs to ward off osteoporosis because calcium needs stomach acid to be absorbed well. Yet, many of those who desperately need calcium, those over 60, have reduced amounts of natural stomach acid.

THE VINEGAR DIET

Traditionally, a teaspoon each of vinegar and honey are taken with a full glass of water 30 minutes before the two largest meals of the day. Taken this way they help control appetite, aid digestion and supply trace amounts of a spectacular number of nutrients. (If you take a vinegar tonic on a daily basis, use a straw so tooth enamel is protected.)

Lose weight, safely, with vinegar.

The secret to the vinegar diet is proportion!! Each time you eat, use the drawing on the opposite page. It shows you how much of each food group to eat at each meal. It is essential to use these proportions every time you eat! Every day, you need to include foods in your diet from all five food groups:

Grains & breads - includes rice, potatoes, pasta, beans, baked goods
Vegetables - includes broccoli, squash, green beans, corn, tomatoes
Fruits - includes oranges, bananas, grapes, pears, berries, melons
Proteins - includes meat, fish, peanut butter, beans
Dairy - includes milk, yogurt, cottage cheese, buttermilk

If you are eating a big meal and heap up lots of food on the bread and grain section, then you must also heap up lots of food on all the other sections. This way, the food you eat stays in proper proportion. If you go back for seconds, you must eat some of each food group, in the proportions shown. If you are only eating a snack, fill each section only partially. Add fats and sweets sparingly to the foods above and drink six to eight glasses of water a day. To maintain an average weight and to get the nutrients your body needs each day, you need:

THE VINEGAR DIET

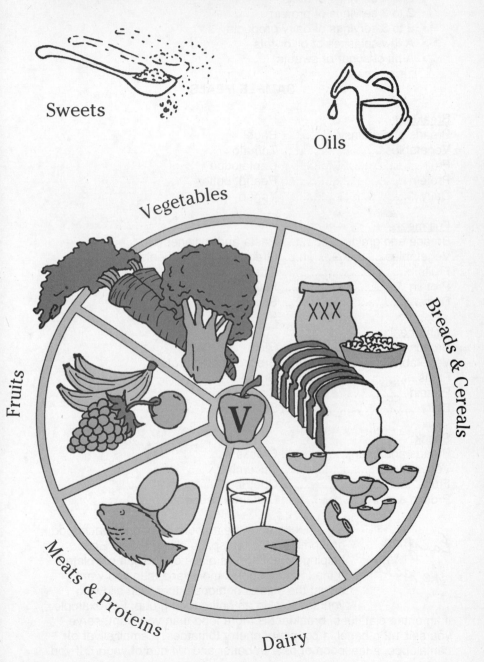

Sweets

Oils

Vegetables

Fruits

Breads & Cereals

Meats & Proteins

Dairy

- 6 to 11 servings of breads and grains
- 3 to 5 servings of vegetables
- 2 to 4 servings of fruits
- 2 to 3 servings of protein
- 2 to 3 servings of dairy products
- A few splashes of oil or fats
- A bit of sugar or sweets

SAMPLE MEALS

Breakfast:
Breads and grains .... Bagel
Vegetables............................ Tomato
Fruit .... Cantaloupe
Protein .... Peanut butter
Dairy .... Yogurt

Full meal:
Breads and grains .... Pasta and a dinner roll
Vegetables............................ Green beans and beets
Fruits..................................... Orange
Protein .... Fish
Dairy .... Skim milk

Light meal:
Breads and grains .... Rice
Vegetables............................ Broccoli and carrots
Fruits..................................... Grapes
Protein .... Chicken
Dairy .... Skim milk

Snack:
Breads and grains .... Crackers
Vegetables............................ Cucumber
Fruits..................................... Cherries
Protein & dairy...................... Cottage cheese

Easy on the salt.

Make sure the amount of food for each food group fits inside the space allotted for it. Each helping must fit on its place on the sample plate. If the total amount is more food than you want, adjust the size of portions rather than allowing yourself to skip an entire food group. For example, if an entire plateful of breakfast is more food than you want, serve yourself 1/2 a bagel, a couple of cherry tomatoes, a small sliver of cantaloupe, a teaspoon of peanut butter and 1/4 cup of yogurt. If you want a hearty breakfast, serve yourself an entire bagel, a large tomato, 1/2 a cantaloupe, a tablespoon of peanut butter and a cup of yogurt. Occasionally, one section of a meal may overlap another. When this happens, make up for it at the next meal. For example, if a piece of fish overlaps its section at one meal, you may skip the protein section on the next meal and fill that area with extra vegetables or fruits. And remember, many kinds of beans can do double duty because they are good sources of protein.

Keep fats and oils to a minimum by trimming meats and avoiding fried foods. Limit sugar and sweets by replacing them with fruits. Fortified vinegars can help you increase the amount of vegetable and fruit nutrients you get. They are also good ways to get your daily servings of vinegar. For example, in the sample full meal, serve the fish topped with lemon or garlic fortified vinegar. In the sample snack, apple fortified vinegar is a smooth, tasty way to add flavor, nutrients and excitement to the cottage cheese.

COLOR MATTERS

Good food comes in a healthy rainbow of colors. Always look at your plate of food and check that you have included many different colors. If the plate is mostly white, faded and colorless your food is probably over-processed and short of nutrients. Your diet should be a joyful mix of color. Check for a variety of colors at every meal, every day. Include foods that are red, orange, yellow, purple and green because:

Red foods can contain lycopene that fights cancer; others have beta-cyanin that fights bacteria. Red foods include radishes, tomatoes, strawberries, cherries, raspberries, grapes, peppers, beans, watermelon, cranberries, beets and apples.
Orange foods can contain beta carotene, which lowers the risk of getting some cancers. Orange foods include squash, carrots, oranges, pumpkins, sweet potatoes, cantaloupe, papayas and apricots.
Yellow foods can contain lutein to help preserve eyesight by fighting macular degeneration. Others have the antioxidant anthoxanthin, or an anti-inflammatory, antibacterial and antiviral substance called quercetin. Yellow foods include raspberries, cherries, peppers, grapefruit, squash, lemons, corn, beans, bananas, pineapple and apples.
Purple foods can contain anthocyanin, a phytochemical that attacks free radicals while also dilating blood vessels to reduce the risk of stroke and heart attack. Purple foods include egg plant, red cabbage, blackberries, raspberries, grapes, blueberries, cherries and plums.
Green foods can contain indoles that block some cancer causing chemicals. Green foods include broccoli, Brussels sprouts, kiwis,

grapes, peppers, spinach, beans, apples, asparagus, celery, kale, okra and cucumbers.

BOOST THE HEALTH EFFECTS OF THE VINEGAR DIET!

You can multiply the benefits of my vinegar diet by drinking six to eight glasses of water each day and limiting coffee to one or two cups. Take an energy boosting mini vacation of 10 minutes from your usual day. Get outside into the fresh air. Move around a bit; let your mind wander. Never skip meals. Eat several small meals instead of one or two large ones that can make you feel sluggish and bloated. Give yourself a new routine by making changes in the way you do things during the day.

To the body most "diets" seem like a deadly famine.

Learn to reward yourself in nonfood ways. Have a massage instead of dinner at a fancy restaurant. You will feel better, longer. Do some deep breathing exercises instead of eating a handful of cookies. Move around more to improve circulation. Wear brightly colored, soft comforting clothes. Sit in the sunshine, outside when the weather is nice, at a window when weather is bitter. But most important, begin right this minute! Put a smile on your face, think about something pleasant, and vow to yourself that you are going to begin eating for health with the next bite you take by following the vinegar diet plan!

Vinegar does even more. One of biggest jobs vinegar does in the human body is promote the growth of beneficial bacteria. They are needed to keep disease-producing germs at bay. For example, human intestines contain millions of good bacteria (such as bifidus and lactobicillus) to keep the gastrointestinal tract healthy and disease free. Helpful bacteria in the intestines also work to:

Support the immune system
Help digest food
Make some vitamins
Keep the intestines acidic
Discourage illness caused by E. coli and clostridia bacteria

Fruits and vegetables are storehouses of flavonoids, biflavonoids and carotenoids. These are wondrous antioxidants with the ability to neutralize free radicals that age the body. Of the hundreds of flavonoids in plants, more than 60 kinds (such as beta carotene) have been found in the foods we eat. For example, you can get your entire daily beta carotene needs in half a cantaloupe or half a carrot. The cantaloupe has the vitamin C of two small oranges.

Cholesterol

Almost all body cells have some cholesterol. The body makes some, and it is found in all animal-based foods. Meat, fish, poultry, eggs and dairy products all have it. Some cholesterol is essential. The body uses it to build new cells, make hormones and as an aid in digestion. Too much contributes to clogging arteries and heart damage. Vegetables, which are cholesterol free, are a very healthy way to get protein. Cold water fish help maintain low cholesterol, too. They bring cholesterol lowering omega-3 fatty acids to the body. (This is probably because of the way omega-3 fatty acids act on platelet aggregation and lipid metabolism.)

Fiber

Vegetables and fruits bring fiber to the diet. Fiber helps regulate digestion, absorbs cholesterol and dilutes toxins that cause cancer. Foods containing soluble fiber include rye, oats, legumes and fruits such as apples. Food containing insoluble fiber include whole wheat, bran and most fruits and vegetables.

Carbohydrates

High doses of sugar hurts cells' ability to fight disease. Complex carbohydrates in fruits and vegetables stay in the digestive system longer, and are fed into the blood stream more slowly than refined sugars. This slow, steady digestion keeps essential nutrients in the bloodstream. They bathe cells in healing antioxidants for long periods of time. A cell which is bathed in nutrients will go a long way in healing itself. A low fat, sugar and cholesterol diet may be helpful in fighting infection. So is eating enough protein. The risk of many chronic diseases of elder years is increased by poor eating habits in younger years. And poor nutrition makes recovery from illness take longer.

Thermogenesis — A Word You Need To Know

Thermogenesis is the process by which the body turns food into energy. This energy is used to warm the body, make muscles work and power the brain. And, some is used to repair and replace worn out tissue. When you eat, think about what kind of nutrients that particular food is giving your body. If it is a very fatty food it may supply more energy than the body can work off, without giving it the vitamins and minerals it needs to repair injury. The result is fat added to the body.

When fat is burned to make heat it is called thermogenesis.

93

Common Food Myths
There are no calories in cottage cheese
Pickles and milk at the same meal will make you sick
Bread sticks have very few calories
Brown eggs are better than white eggs
Ice cream is the secret to losing weight
Hot food is healthier than cold food

Good health and a youthful appearance go hand in hand with a good diet. It has been said that the body's real age is tied closer to the health of its immune system than to its calendar age. I believe nutritious food and moderate exercise are the best ways to empower the immune system, to bring a healthy glow to your face and to put a spring into your step. You can improve your appearance by feeding your body everything it needs. This includes eating a wide variety of foods. Promise yourself you will begin today to make better choices.

Is The Vinegar Diet For You?
Ask your doctor before beginning any changes to your usual diet. The suggestions offered in *THE VINEGAR DIET* may be appropriate for healthy adults — they are not intended for children, the frail elderly, those taking medications or with chronic health conditions — without the approval of a medical professional!

Can Vinegar Melt Away Pounds And Inches?
Doctors tell us when calories are restricted as a way to lose weight 95% of diets fail! Harsh dieting, with strict calorie reduction, is harmful to the body and an unnatural process. When you are hungry the natural thing to do is eat! Strict "dieting" can affect the immune system, making it unable to do a good job fighting off disease. People who spend a lifetime gradually putting on pounds should not expect to take it all off overnight.

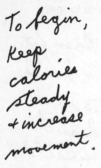

To begin, Keep calories steady + increase movement.

CAN YOU REALLY MELT FAT AWAY?

YES! There is a way for you to eat all the food you need to feel full and create the slimmer body you have always wanted! If weight loss makes you look drawn and ill you are losing weight too fast. Losing weight is a very complex process. You can win the war against unwanted pounds, but it is important to not lose important nutrients along with the weight. What is the very best diet of all? The one that works for you — the vinegar diet plan! It can help you keep off unwanted pounds for life. Its slow and steady weight loss means you never need to 'go on a diet' again. You will feel better about yourself and have more energy from the very beginning. It

THE VINEGAR WEIGHT LOSS DIET

Sweets

Oils

Vegetables

Fruits

Breads & Cereals

V

Meats & Proteins

Dairy

is a way of living, a plan for a healthier life!

How To Be Thinner, Look Younger, Feel More Vigorous! Depriving yourself of food, being constantly hungry or even having to count calories is not the way to create a healthy new body.

Do Not Eat Less Without A Doctor's Supervision! Limiting fat is the simplest way to control weight. As a bonus, you decrease the risk of stroke, high blood pressure and diabetes. Your goal, for the most successful, longest lasting weight loss is to begin your vinegar diet by keeping the number of calories you eat each day about the same as you are eating right now. Simply switch fat calories to calories from fruits and vegetables and begin to increase the amount of exercise you get.

SAMPLE DIET MEALS

Breakfast:
Breads and grains .... Puffed wheat
Vegetables................................. Tomato
Fruit .... Cantaloupe
Protein .... Slice of turkey breast
Dairy .... Skim milk

Full meal:
Breads and grains .... Sweet potato
Vegetables................................. Green beans, beets, salad
Fruits.. Orange, kiwi
Protein .... Fish
Dairy .... Skim milk

Light meal:
Breads and grains .... Rice
Vegetables................................. Broccoli, carrots
Fruits.. Grapes, apple
Protein .... Chicken
Dairy .... Yogurt

Snack:
Breads and grains .... Crackers
Vegetables................................. Cucumber, celery
Fruits.. Cherries, grapefruit
Protein & dairy........................... Cottage cheese

Make sure the size of each helping of food fits on its place on the sample plate. Compared to my standard vinegar diet, the vinegar weight loss diet gives you slightly smaller portions of breads and grains and slightly larger portions of vegetables and fruits. The protein and dairy sections are exactly the same. If the diet seems to offer more food than you want, adjust the size of portions rather than skip an entire food group. For example, if breakfast is more food than you want to eat, serve yourself 1/2 cup of cereal, a couple of cherry tomatoes, a small sliver of cantaloupe, a very small piece of turkey and a glass of skim milk. If you are very hungry, serve yourself a full cup of cereal, a large tomato, 1/2 a cantaloupe, a small slice of turkey and drink a full glass of skim milk.

If a food does overlap one section, make it up at the next meal. For example, if a piece of fish overlaps its section at one meal, you may skip the protein section at the next meal and fill that area with extra vegetables or fruits.

Lose Pounds – The Vinegar Way
As you can see, the vinegar weight loss diet is very similar to the regular vinegar diet. And that is the magic of this eating plan! You lose weight by eating extra vegetables and fruits and increasing how much you move around. This makes it an amazing – perhaps the ultimate – weapon against fat!

You will protect the health of your heart and arteries, and lose weight, by eating very small amounts of fats and oils. Limit sugars and sweets, too. Use fortified vinegars to increase the amount of vegetable and fruit nutrients you get, and as an alternative to drinking vinegar in water. For example, in the sample breakfast the cantaloupe is delicious topped with fortified raspberry vinegar. In the sample light meal fortified carrot vinegar can be served over the broccoli. Or, spoon warm garlic fortified vinegar over both the broccoli and carrots. Several times a week substitute legumes, such as beans, for animal sources of protein. You will eliminate cholesterol loaded fats and be able to eat much larger portions for the same calories. To use the plate diagram for plant-based sources of protein (such as beans) use both the bread and grain and protein sections when filling your plate.

Thermogenesis — A Concept For Losing Weight
The body thinks of food as fuel. So, its first instinct is to turn it into energy. Some energy is used to power muscles and the brain. A lot of energy is used to heat the body and a tiny bit is used to replace worn out or damaged cells. Only after doing all this does the body make fat. If there is a sudden reduction in the amount of food the body gets it panics and thinks a famine has started. To protect itself from dying in this famine all available calories are turned into fat. And, worst of all, the body sends urgent signals of hunger to its appetite control

center.

Little wonder many doctors tell us nearly all of the weight lost by conventional calorie reduction 'dieting' is soon regained! The very best way to begin a weight loss program is to lower total body fat and increase lean body mass, while keeping actual weight steady. Muscle takes more calories to maintain, even at rest. This means the body uses more calories, so weight is gradually reduced, even though the amount of food eaten stays constant.

This thermogenic weight loss happens because muscles have a higher metabolic rate than fat. And, muscles weigh more than fat for the same bulk. So, for the same total weight, extra muscle means a slimmer body. And, increased muscle tone will enable you to have a firmer abdomen and stronger back muscles, which will make you appear slimmer. As more and more fat is replaced with muscle, the higher metabolic rate will need enough extra calories that the body will begin using up its stored fat.

The second part of thermogenic weight loss is based on the fact that the body's biggest use of calories is to make heat. What is left over goes to fix worn out body parts and allow muscles to do work. Only after all this is fat produced. If the cycle is interrupted anywhere along the way, there is no fat to store.

Thermogenesis, turning food into heat, can be increased by diet choices. You can feel it begin when you eat a big meal and your body gets hot as it burns food. Some foods do this longer and better than others. They encourage the body to burn calories faster by increasing metabolism. By adding these foods to the diet and by moving around more you lose weight without reducing the total number of calories in the diet. Healthy, fat-free fortified vinegars (like all foods) get the process of thermogenesis to begin working for you.

If you suddenly restrict calories, the body slows down its metabolic rate. Food is stored as fat instead of being used as energy. When the rate of metabolism is high, more food is burned and less is available to make fat. (When the rate of metabolism is very low it is almost impossible to lose weight, even on a severely restricted calorie diet.) Cold, food and exercise speed up thermogenesis. Increasing the number of calories the body burns is a sure, safe and lasting way to lose weight.

Cold makes the body work harder and burn more calories to keep warm. That is why I believe cooling off the body helps increase its metabolic rate. For example, always wearing a heavy sweater could help the body stay fat by reducing the amount of calories it needs to burn to stay warm.

Exercise turns up the body's fat-burning metabolism. This faster burning of calories continues for hours after exercise has ended. For this reason I suggest spreading exercise out over the entire day, rather than limiting it to a single session. To practice this, get moving early in the day. Make your body wake up and begin using calories as soon as possible. Follow up with frequent short exercise periods.

Food such as capsicum-containing peppers increase metabolism. They burn off more calories than they contain because they stimulate the body. Thermogenic agents such as hot peppers and chili powder also have lots of vitamins C and E, carotenes and antioxidants. They even have substances to fight the bacteria that causes some diarrhea. Fennel is another good "diet" food. Fennel can be of great help in a weight loss program because it helps tone and stimulate the gastro-intestinal system and reduces the gas that can be produced by a diet high in vegetables and fruits.

MY SECRET TO LOSING WEIGHT

The real secret to losing unwanted pounds and inches is to get the body to increase the amount of fuel it burns without sending it into panic anti-famine mode. To do this it needs a reasonable amount of many kinds of food and an adequate amount of exercise. Exercise need not be strenuous. Walking is one of the very best ways to exercise. When you eat healthy and move around a bit, your weight tends to take care of itself!

Danger In Reducing Calories

Calorie restriction diets usually cause the loss of important muscle tissue as well as fat. The ratio can be significant. For many dieters, half of their weight loss is muscle or bone. Only half of it is the unwanted fat. Even with heavy exercise calorie restriction usually results in at least one-fourth of the weight coming from lean body mass. It is important to eat some protein, as it is an important part of the system that tells your body when to stop eating. Some diets distort the value of protein by encouraging the dieter to eat huge amounts of it. These diets cause the body to lose a lot of water, rapidly. This can make it seem as if there has been a sudden weight loss.

Too much protein can increase the amount of precious calcium lost in the urinary tract and has been linked to more frequent bone fractures. The healthiest way to eat protein is in proper proportion to other food. The protein space on my vinegar diet drawing shows

99

you the proportion of protein the U.S. Department of Agriculture recommends in its Food Guide Pyramid.

Water Washes Away Pounds

Water is especially important when losing weight. Drink at least eight full glasses a day. Coffee, tea and colas do not count as part of this. Extra water helps the body wash away toxins. It also encourages you to eat less. For variety, try water with a twist of lime, a wedge of lemon, a drop of vanilla or a dash of herbal vinegar. When you think you are really hungry it can help to drink a glass of water and wait a few minutes. You may find you are not so hungry after all!

Vinegar Is Essential

Vinegar, as acetic acid, is used by the body in the process by which it burns both carbohydrates and fat. It is naturally present in most plant and animal tissues. The human body even makes it. Vinegar also plays a role in how the body stores fat. When vinegar enters the blood stream it is carried to the kidneys and muscles. There, it either becomes energy or is used to make body tissues through its role in making essential amino acids. It even facilitates the process which forms the red blood cells that supply the body's oxygen!

FAST START TIPS

For a thinner you, melt pounds away safely with vinegar. When you follow the vinegar weight loss plan for healthy eating your weight loss may not be sudden, but it will be permanent! You can give up yo-yo dieting that takes off a few pounds one week and puts them back on the next. The vinegar diet encourages you to eat a balanced diet, including food from all five food groups.

Bring out the good taste of these foods with healthy splashes of plain or flavored apple cider vinegar. It has only two calories in an entire tablespoon. Or, increase their nutrient content dramatically with fortified vinegars. If you follow this plan you will not have the overwhelming fatigue that goes with many diet plans. Actually, you should have more energy! Some other ways to get your weight loss program off to a fast start follow:

- Eat a raw vegetable or fruit half an hour before a meal
- Eat only lean meats, and eat them less often
- Add more cold water fish to your diet
- Use small plates to serve your meals
- Stop eating when you are full, even if food remains on your plate
- You do not have to clean up your plate
- Substitute pureed pumpkin or applesauce for half of the fat or oil

in baked goods
- Use only low fat dairy products
- Bake or simmer in no-fat sauces and broil rather than fry
- Eat slowly because it takes about 20 minutes for the body to be able to judge when you are full
- When you really want something you know is not good for you, eat at least one bite. In the long run you will be less likely to pig out on it

MISCELLANEOUS DIETING TIPS

Plants contain thousands of different substances. There is no way a pill can duplicate the exact effect of eating a fresh orange or a ripe tomato. The only way to get all the nutrients needed for a healthy body is to eat a variety of good foods. Regular exercise and enough pure water are also needed. This is a plan that is safe, sure and will bring results that last for life!

Many doctors recommend a daily vitamin and mineral supplement. This is partly because so many of the foods most people eat are so heavily processed. And, it is because so few people eat the five servings of fruits and vegetables recommended for good health. As you make changes in your diet, do a little bit at a time. Use fats sparingly. Remember, all animal fats (and some vegetable fats) are associated with atherosclerosis.

Mushrooms + truffles are in the mold & mildew family!

Do not shock your system with sudden changes in the way you eat or exercise. Strict calorie reduction can cause fatigue, and it makes the body's fat-burning mechanism slow down to conserve fuel. Even good things need to be done gradually! Concentrate on high bulk, high fiber foods rather than concentrated sources of nutrients. For example, mushrooms contain about 60 calories in an entire pound, 25 calories in a cup. They are high in fiber and contain biotin, one of the complex of B vitamins involved in the digestion of fats and proteins. Some of the nutrients in mushrooms are only available to the body when they are cooked. Cooking also deactivates hydrazines in mushrooms that can increase the risk of getting cancer.

Spot Toning
Yes, I believe you can reduce places on your body that are especially troublesome to you! Exercise which tones a particular set of muscles can give the appearance of spot reducing. For example, tummy toning can be achieved by increasing the strength of the

101

abdominal muscles. These stronger muscles will hold a sagging tummy in and up, even if total fat mass stays the same. Strengthening back muscles can help you stand up straight and appear thinner, too.

Fat Makes Fat!

If there is too much fat in your diet your body will use it instead of burning the body fat you want to lose. One way to use less fat is to substitute vinegar-based toppings for fatty sauces and spreads. It also helps to use butter or margarine at room temperature so you can spread it thinner. Apply it with a small spatula and you will use even less! Other ways to cut down on the fat in your diet follow:

FATTY FOOD	BETTER CHOICE
Sour cream	Whipped cottage cheese
Granola	Oatmeal with raisins
Cheese omelet	Egg substitute & vegetables
Beef & cheese nachos	Bean burrito
Fettuccine Alfredo	Spaghetti with tomato sauce
Sweet & sour pork	Pork stir fry
Hamburger, fries, shake	Salad, baked potato, tea
Loaded pizza	Vegetarian pizza
Microwave popcorn	Air-popped popcorn
Danish	Fruit
Whole milk	Skim milk
Deep fried chicken leg	Broiled, skinless chicken breast

LOSE A LITTLE, GAIN A LOT!

Why lose weight? Because even a small weight loss can give you a lot of benefits. Diabetes, high blood pressure, atherosclerosis, heart disease and cancer are all tied to extra body fat. Even a little weight off can decrease risk of osteoarthritis, even in your hands. (Researchers think a chemical in stored fat increases the progression of osteoarthritis.) Where and when you gain matters, too. Extra pounds on your stomach are more serious than weight carried on the hips and thighs. And, if you have gained more than 10 pounds since becoming an adult it is more of a problem than if you have always carried the extra weight. Middle-of-life weight gain is especially dangerous for women. A mere 10 pounds can raise the risk of heart attack by 25%. (25 pounds may triple it!) Gaining weight as an adult tends to increase blood fat, pressure and sugar levels.

Visualization

Put your daydreams to work for you and they will become reality! You can use visualization to reshape your body. It makes any weight reduction program more effective. Some say you can even increase your metabolism this way. Put a picture in your mind of your new thin self. Enjoy the way you feel. Do this before you get out of bed in the morning, during meals and as you drop off to sleep at night. Soon it will be real.

Aromatherapy

Smell is 90% of the body's sensation of taste and researchers are using this to help people lose weight. They have found that, for some people, smelling banana, peppermint or apple fragrance allows them to keep from overeating. Average weight loss using aromatherapy is about a pound a week. These odors probably work by making the body think it has eaten.

Variety! Variety!

We know the body needs a variety of smells and tastes at each meal to satisfy its food cravings. Be sure to include sweet and sour, salty and tangy foods in your diet, along with a range of colors. Experiment at the supermarket with new and different foods. Try a pre-made salad, tiny baby carrots or a prepared selection of vegetables such as broccoli and cauliflower. They may be more expensive than your usual way of buying vegetables, but compared to eating out or a pack-aged 'diet food' meal they are cheap. Their wonderful nutritional benefits are worth it if this is the only way you are going to eat these healthy foods.

The French Connection

Wine and France have an inescapable connection. It is home to some of the great wines of the world. And wine is one of the substances from which an excellent vinegar is made. Wine, like vinegar, is an acidic liquid, much like the chemistry of the body. It has long been recognized as an aid to digestion. Now it is said to do even more! Many believe a small glass of wine with or before meals can have a definite effect on weight. It does this because it seems to reduce the total amount of fuel the body desires. The effect is especially noticeable when compared to the effect of unsweetened liquids. Red grapes, from which red wine vinegar is made, have been found to contain a very special antioxidant. This substance, proanthocyanidin, is extremely effective at fighting free radicals associated with degenerative diseases and aging.

Fasting — Is It For You?

A weight-loss fast is a period of time where only liquids are taken. It can bring about an immediate small amount of weight loss, but because it throws the body into famine protection mode it is of very limited long term value. Weight lost through fasting inevitably returns, often within a day or two. It is not a way to permanently lose weight.

Arthritis sufferers sometimes use a fast to control pain. It has been found that fasting changes immune cells, so some kinds of arthritis may be calmed by a fast. Although fasting may bring temporary relief, it must not be overused. A low fat and protein diet that has lots of vegetables and fruits may work just as well.

If you decide to fast while on the vinegar weight loss diet be sure to supplement the vinegar and honey tonic with large amounts of vegetable and fruit juices. And, keep the fast short. Prolonged fasting can cause serious damage to the body!

Is The Vinegar Weight Loss Diet For You?

Ask your doctor before beginning any changes to your usual diet! Feel free to show your health care provider the drawings that show you how to fill your plate for the vinegar weight loss diet. And please remember —suggestions offered in the vinegar diet may be appropriate for healthy adults — they are not intended for children, the frail elderly, those taking medications or with chronic health conditions — without the approval of a medical professional! I do not recommend fasting to lose weight.

BUILD UP YOUR BODY WITH VINEGAR

THE VINEGAR DIET can help you create the stronger body you have always wanted! With its help I feel you can gain strength, energy and vigor. It can be a healthy beginning for building up a frail, too thin, undermuscled or flabby body. If you are underweight or disabled, you – most of all – need the nutrients of vegetables, fruits and whole grains. Use the drawing every time you eat. It shows you how much of each food group to eat at each meal.

It is essential to use these proportions every time you eat! The secret to building up your body with the vinegar diet is proportion!! Every day, you need to include foods in your diet from all five food groups. Add healthy oils for extra calories and smooth taste, fortified vinegars for concentrated nutrients, a few sweets to perk up your taste buds and drink six to eight glasses of water a day. To maintain an average weight and to get the nutrients your body needs each day, you need:

6 to 11 servings of breads and grains
3 to 5 servings of vegetables
2 to 4 servings of fruits
2 to 3 servings of protein
2 to 3 servings of dairy products

Many older adults, particularly those who live alone, are at risk for becoming too thin. If body weight is too low the immune system may not be getting all the nutrients it needs to keep the body healthy. Frequent colds and bouts of flu, having several allergies, slow healing of cuts and scrapes and being tired every day could mean you have a weak immune system. Because very low body weight can lead to greater susceptibility to disease, if you are thin it is extra-important to eat some food, each day, from each food group.

fat has 9 calories per gram, protein and carbo-hydrates have 4.

To build up your body, choose foods with concentrated calories and nutrients. Eat bananas Instead of grapes, avocados rather than watermelon, corn or beets rather than lettuce or mushrooms. All beans are good for you because they are rich sources of the protein you need to build up a damaged or frail body. You may tolerate small meals every three hours better than three large meals.

Fats are the most concentrated fuel for your body, as well as being an essential part of the taste, flavor and texture of food. For the same bulk, fat has more than twice the calories of other food. Because saturated fats, such as those from meats, may be associated with a higher risk of clogged arteries, choose healthy vegetable oils. Hazelnut, walnut and flaxseed oils are good choices for mixing with vinegars. So are monounsaturated corn, safflower and soy oils. For cooking, use oils that are resistant to heat, such as canola or olive.

Exercise is as important for normalizing weight as diet! It increases energy and lifts your mood. Your first goal should be to increase endurance and flexibility. To begin, stand up straight and breath deeply. Get oxygen flowing to all parts of your body. Short walks throughout the day help do this. Regular, gentle exercise will increase the body's ability to move and bend and firm up flabby muscles. Begin by doing several repeats of light exercises, rather than trying to do heavy exercises too soon.

Twenty minutes of exercise, three times a week can add years to your life. It is not necessary to do all 20 minutes at once. It is often better to start out exercising a few minutes at a time, spread out during the day. When physical problems slow you down exercise may seem like the last thing you need to do. Actually, it is probably more important for those with physical problems to exercise than for others. Move the parts of the body that you can. If you use a walker or cane, you still need to move your body as much as possible to retain balance and coordination. Do a lot of stretching and range of motion exercises to keep joints mobile.

Exercise is needed for bones to retain their calcium. Only a small part of the body's total calcium circulates in the blood, so tests can show a blood level that is normal, even when the bones are honeycombed by loss of calcium. Mild exercise is especially important for those with fibromyalgia or any other type of arthritis. Gentle exercise is needed to strengthen tendons and ligaments around joints. Those with mild high blood pressure may find exercise lowers it into normal range.

Is The Best Way To Fitness Too Easy?
The President's Council on Physical Fitness and Sports calls walking the slower, surer way to fitness! Walking burns about the same number of calories as running, for the same distance. The best news of all is that the less you weigh, the fewer calories you burn and the more you weigh, the more calories you burn in this easiest of exercises. Many researchers believe walking is better than running for overall body conditioning. For best results swing your arms while you walk. It is also a good idea to do stretching exercises at the beginning and end of your walk. Take it slowly at first. If walking makes you too breathless to talk, you are going too fast. Getting some exercise is more important than how fast you go or how far. The biggest benefits come when those who do not usually exercise begin moving. Advantages to walking for exercise include:

- No lessons are needed, almost everyone can do it without training
  - You can do it most any time, anywhere
  - It is free
  - No special equipment is needed

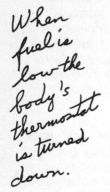

Expensive sports drinks are unnecessary. A teaspoon each of vinegar and honey stirred into a quart of water makes a good substitute. Or, plain water will do fine! Exercise tends to normalize appetite. The body goes on burning more fuel for hours after exercise. Firm, healthy muscles burn more fuel, even at rest, than soft, flabby fat. Exercise and the extra nutrition of fortified vinegar can aid in lowering cholesterol, boost the immune system, restore age-wasted muscles and more.

Fatigue
Chronic fatigue is not a natural part of aging. It is a sign

something is wrong, perhaps that the immune system is not functioning at its peak level. To find out why you are overly tired, decide when it happens most. Keep a chart for a week and write down the time you are really tired each day. Then, look back and see how this relates to your eating habits. Be especially aware of your use of caffeine, too. It may increase fatigue symptoms. Low levels of the B complex of vitamins reduces endurance and results in feelings of tiredness.

Using music to help energize your body and lift your mood may also help. You may need to add a protein, carbohydrate and calcium rich snack for an afternoon energy boost. Cheese and crackers, with a rich honey and strawberry fortified vinegar to dip them in tastes great. Or, try a slice of chicken on half an English muffin and a spoonful of cooked prunes drizzled with cucumber-celery fortified vinegar. Wash it down with skim milk. A short afternoon nap may help, too. If you are very thin, use the principals of thermogenesis and help the body conserve heat. Be sure to wear a heavy sweater when it is cool so the body does not need to burn a lot of calories to stay warm. Fight fatigue by eating healthy food, getting daily exercise and taking an active interest in the world around you.

RECIPES FOR SUCCESS

You can normalize your weight without drugs.

If weight is a problem, you need a better way of eating, not another diet! We have come a long way from the days when it was thought food left on the table overnight fed the fairies, thus ensuring good fortune for the household. We now know it is the cook who shapes the fortunes of the household by preparing healthy food! The rich, vivid taste sensation of fortified vinegar can help stimulate an appetite which has become dulled with age or depression. Vegetables have fiber, vitamins and minerals. They are low in salt and most are fat-free. Beta-carotene rich vegetables fight colon, lung, bladder and esophagus cancer. A special carotenoid (lutein) fights deterioration of the retina. All foods with soluble fiber, such as the apples used to make apple cider vinegar, are good for preventing heart disease.

Recipe Tips
Get meals off to a healthy start with homemade soup. Good choices include chicken, celery, pumpkin and vegetable. In clear soups, use the liquid from canned vegetables or the water used to cook fresh ones. It can contain nearly one-third of the total nutrients. Pep up mild chicken soup with a splash of herbal vinegar or a bit of fortified garlic vinegar. Rinse cooked meats for soups (such as hamburger) in water

107

to remove their fat. Prepare healthy cream soups by using skim milk made with twice the normal milk powder.

Use mustard, ketchup or apple butter on breads and rolls instead of fatty spreads. Better yet, drizzle them with fortified vinegar or cottage cheese blended with apple cider vinegar.

Cook stuffing outside a chicken or turkey to avoid the risk of salmonella germs. As a bonus, it will be lower in calories than the exact same stuffing cooked inside fowl! (If cooked in the bird, stuffing soaks up melted fat.) For a healthy change try white or brown rice instead of bread for stuffing. Use tomatoes, corn, mushrooms and red and green peppers, too.

Cream cheese is a fatty food!

Skip the salt in boiling pasta and vegetables. Substitute a splash of apple cider or herbal vinegar.

Make lighter corn muffins and brownies by replacing half the oil with applesauce, mashed pumpkin or sweet potato.

An easy, tasty dessert can be made by baking bananas, pears or apples with cinnamon and nutmeg.

Add a bit of peppermint to salads for a fresh taste. It is said to sharpen the memory and stimulate circulation.

Skim milk tastes better with a tablespoon or so of dry milk stirred into each glass. A dash of vanilla or honey makes it even better. Add dry skim milk to mashed potatoes, cooked cereal, gravy, ground meats, casseroles, and baked goods to increase the amount of calcium you eat. Be sure to finish the milk at the bottom of the cereal bowl because many nutrients dissolve into it.

For a fruity milk treat mix 3/4 cup very cold skim milk, 1/4 cup frozen orange juice concentrate and 1/4 cup crushed ice.

Croissants + muffins are weighty food!

The FDA warns that those who take many of the prescription appetite suppressants increase their risk of developing primary pulmonary hypertension by as much as 20 times. Diarrhea, dizziness, memory lapses and depression are common short-term side effects of weight loss drugs. Long term studies on safety and effectiveness have not yet been completed. A nonprescription supplement, chromium picolinate, seems to have fewer known side effects than some other weight loss agents; but there have been no long term tests to confirm this. And, it has not been proven effective for most people.

Caffeine is the most popular stimulant drug in the world! Until 1991 caffeine was used in over-the-counter weight loss products. The FDA no longer permits this, as it as been deemed to have no long term effect on weight. Colas, regular tea, coffee and chocolate contain caffeine. Caffeine increases metabolism, especially when combined with aspirin. Unfortunately it also encourages brittle bones. It is estimated that one six ounce cup of coffee pulls about five milligrams of calcium from the body. Replacing this calcium takes the equivalent of the concentrated power of two tablespoons of yogurt. Cafestol and kahweol are in the oils in ground coffee. They are not in instant or filtered drip coffee, but remain in percolated coffee. Drinking even four cups a day of oil-containing coffee may significantly increase the risk of heart disease.

One thing all weight loss drugs share is that when they are stopped, any weight lost tends to be regained! Considering their many, often dangerous, side effects they are a poor substitute for a healthy diet and exercise. All weight loss drugs carry some health warnings. Vegetables, fruits and whole grains do not. Whenever a product has dangers attached to it, proceed with great caution. You may not need to take that risk. The vinegar diet, with its use of fortified vinegars to add all the goodness of vegetables and fruits to your diet may be what you need.

No matter what scientists finally decide about vinegar's usefulness in the diet, people have instinctively felt, for untold centuries, that vinegar was good for them. It is truly a living substance, capable of bringing health benefits far beyond the ability of today's medical world to fully comprehend! Vinegar can be of great value in a weight loss program; enriched vinegars are especially helpful. Fortified vinegars are a fat-free way to increase fiber, vitamins and minerals in the diet without multiplying calories; tasty carrier for substances that can actually burn away body fat; healthy way to satisfy cravings by indulging the way mature taste buds function.

Each one of the tongue's nearly 10,000 individual taste buds is made up of a cluster of microscopic cells arranged around a tiny pore that collects saliva. The tongue can only detect substances which are dissolved in saliva. If the mouth is overly dry, the sensation of taste is diminished. And, sensitivity to tastes fades as the body ages. Young adults replace their taste buds about once a week. By about 45 years the tongue begins to lose taste buds, because the replacement rate slows. By recognizing the fainter response of the mature tasting system, vinegar can be used to awaken taste buds and provoke responses that make dieting more acceptable to the senses.

Capsicin is a member of the night-shade family

Capsicin (cayenne) peppers probably originated in South America, taking their name from the city that was once the capital of French Guiana. More than 90 kinds of peppers trace their origins to capsicin. These tiny hot peppers have always had a large following that believed they were a healthy food, but new research is showing them to be better than anyone could have imagined! Hot pepper vinegar is a staple in kitchens across the world, one of the simplest ways to add their goodness to the diet. Exciting news about its health benefits has recently been announced by both medical doctors and food researchers. Some of the healthy benefits its use can bring follow:

- Hot peppers can boost the body's metabolic rate (the rate at which it burns calories).
- One-fifth of an ounce of hot pepper vinegar's cayenne can burn away as many as 76 more calories than it contains.
- Hot pepper vinegar causes blood to come to the surface of the body and stimulates it to sweat. This cools the body in hot weather.
- The cayenne in pepper vinegar encourages the adrenal glands to produce cortisone, a natural anti-inflammatory.

As long ago as the time of the ancient Greeks, fennel seeds were popular as an aid to losing weight. Even today, no one is exactly sure why - or how - they work. Many researchers feel their virtues are linked to substances they contain which react in the body much like estrogen. We do know they contain at least 18 different amino acids, 7 minerals (including generous amounts of potassium and calcium), several vitamins (including lots of vitamin A). In addition, their fatty acids are mostly monounsaturated and polyunsaturated (the good kinds). One way to add fennel's flavonoids, vitamins A and C, calcium, phosphorus and potassium to vinegar's goodness is with this dressing: add 10 peppercorns and 3 tablespoons fennel seeds to a pint of white wine vinegar. Let set for at least 2 weeks, then mix with 1 pint water and use on salads.

Apple cider vinegar is helpful in melting away excess pounds. Simply drink a glass of warm water, with a single teaspoon of apple cider vinegar stirred in, before each meal. It moderates the over-robust appetite and melts away fat. Now, whether vinegar actually burns up fatty calories, reins in the over-lusty inclination for partaking of provisions, or simply fills one up with tart vinegar-water, the results are the same. You eat less and the pounds melt away!

Lose Weight The Tasty Way

Vinegar, every day, is not for everyone. Many of my readers tell me vinegar is a tasty, beneficial, addition to their diets. Occasionally, a reader tells me the extra acid causes them some discomfort. YOU SHOULD NEVER CONTINUE EATING ANY FOOD THAT CAUSES DISCOMFORT WITHOUT DISCUSSING IT WITH YOUR HEALTH CARE PROVIDER! The beauty of my vinegar diet plan is that the principles of healthy eating, and the plate templates which show you how to eat foods in proportion to each other, can be used even if vinegar cannot be a regular part of your diet.

If you expect vinegar to aid health, for goodness sake use the good stuff.

Are You Overfed & Undernourished?

An ancient proverb assures us "Diet cures more than doctors." Combine this age-old wisdom with the importance of vinegar and you have — the vinegar diet! My vinegar diet brings together the goodness of vinegar and eating habits needed for continuing health. I believe the balance of food in the vinegar diet furnishes your body with what it needs to resist disease and be vital and vigorous well into old age.

The Vinegar Diet Is Sound Nutrition

Basics of the vinegar diet have been followed by health conscious individuals for decades. What is new, is scientific confirmation that there is a direct association between food and specific diseases. Substances in foods are now linked with arthritis and rheumatism, asthma, allergies, colds and flu, Alzheimer's Disease, diabetes, blood pressure, cancer, heart and cardiovascular disease. Improper eating habits can lead to a depressed immune system and even to more rapid aging! Twenty-five national health and aging organizations, including the American Dietetic Association, National Council on the Aging and American Academy of Family Physicians issued a report on Medical Nutrition Therapy. They propose using foods as medical treatment because many elders' eating habits put them at risk for malnutrition. They suggest preventive health care in the form of nutritional intervention would result in an older population with better immune function, resulting in fewer medical complications; shorter hospital stays; more elders being able to live independently, in their own homes; savings of more than 100 million dollars a year in medical expenses.

Cooking With Vinegar

*V*inegar's introduction to the kitchen was simultaneous with the discovery of wine, more than 10,000 years ago. Through the ages it has added desperately needed nutrients to the meager diets of the poor and delighted the taste buds of the rich. Its ability to break down protein makes it a practical way to tenderize; its preservative qualities offer protection against food poisoning and its antibiotic qualities help protect against illness. Vinegar even plays an important part in developing the texture of baked goods!

Hundreds of foods make use of the preservative and unique taste qualities of vinegar. It is an important part of naturally formed aged cheeses and wine. It is an essential ingredient in catsup and mayonnaise, and is one of the original preservatives for meats and eggs. People have instinctively known, for untold centuries, that vinegar is good for them. It is truly a living substance, capable of bringing health benefits far beyond the ability of today's medical world to fully comprehend.

Throughout the ancient world, cultures depended on the virtues of vinegar to keep them healthy. History tells us the Greeks and Romans often cooked foods in mixtures of honey and vinegar, creating the classic sweet and sour taste celebrated in so many dishes today. They also used vinegar to preserve fruits and vegetables. History reveals a long-standing faith and trust in vinegar-based foods and remedies.

A splash of protein, a dash of carbohydrate, and lots of vitamins and minerals - that's vinegar! A vinegary person is thought of as one who is ill-natured and sour. A vinegary food is apt to be one that has been changed from ordinary to gourmet. Vinegar's unique flavor perks up the taste of foods and keeps them safe from bacteria. Vinegar comes in dozens of kinds and flavors. Some ways to make and use flavored vinegars follow, along with a few other interesting vinegar facts and recipes:

- Vinegar's acid softens muscle fiber in meat so it is tenderized. It also works on fish such as salmon, lobster and oysters. Because meat fiber is broken down and tenderized by vinegar, less expensive cuts can be used in most recipes. They are healthier, since these are the cuts with the least fat.

- Vinegar helps digest tough cellulose, so use it on coarse, fibrous or stringy cooked vegetables such as beets, cabbage, spinach, lettuce and celery. Sprinkle it on raw vegetables such as cucumbers, kale, lettuce, carrots and broccoli.

- Splash vinegar into bean soups, or use herb vinegar on pasta or bean salads to give robust flavor without salt.

- The high acid content reacts with some metals, such as aluminum and iron. It is better to use enamel, glass, or stainless steel pans.

Vinegar is a familiar ingredient in all sorts of condiments. Tomato ketchup, alone, uses up 10% of all the vinegar made in North America. Vinegar also adds its zip to salad dressing, mayonnaise, and a variety of sauces. It is used to make pickles and to preserve foods ranging from beets to eggs to fish.

Osteoporosis is prevented and fought by adding calcium to the diet. Magnesium is also important, because it boosts bone density. Apple cider vinegar contains both and is very good at conveying nutrients from one food to another. Just as the chemicals in cayenne peppers and fennel seeds end up in vinegar, calcium in chicken bones leaches into vinegar during cooking. Use vinegar in many ways in the kitchen, including as an aid in fighting osteoporosis.

TASTE BUDS

Good, sour, acidy vinegar causes saliva to flow. This increases our ability to taste and enjoy other foods. It also aids digestion. Try rubbing a pill you know is bitter on just the center of your tongue. There is no sensation of bitterness because the middle of the tongue has no taste buds. Next, rub the pill across the tip of the tongue and along the edges to sense its true taste.

Foods seasoned with Vinegar taste better.

Each one of the tongue's nearly 10,000 individual taste buds is made up of a cluster of microscopic cells arranged around a tiny pore that collects saliva. The tongue can only detect substances which are dissolved in saliva. So, if the mouth is overly dry, the sensation of taste is diminished. Sensitivity to tastes fades as the body ages. Young adults replace their taste buds about once a week but by about 45 years the tongue begins to lose taste buds. A quality vinegar has a sour taste, without being bitter. By recognizing the fainter response of the mature tasting system, vinegar can be used to awaken taste buds and provoke responses that make dieting more acceptable to the senses.

One reason vinegar is a safe basic ingredient for pickling, marinating and preserving is because it prevents the growth of botulism bacteria. And, at only two calories per tablespoon, it is the ideal topping for salads and vegetables. Vinegar is well-known for its ability to tenderize meat and vegetables and to give foods robust flavor without added salt. It is an inexpensive way to turn dull vegetables into pickled delights and to pep up salads, sauces and dressings. A few ways to use this wondrous fluid alone, or combined with other healthful foods follow. They integrate the latest findings of medical food researchers with the wisdom of traditional healing ways.

Chef's Fish

After deep frying fish, spray each piece, while hot, with a mist of apple cider vinegar. It makes a tangy difference everyone will love and moderates fishy odors. Make strongly flavored fish taste milder by pre-soaking raw fish in 1 cup of water with 1/2 cup white vinegar added to it.

Better Hot Dogs

Improve the flavor of hot dogs by boiling them a few minutes in water with a tablespoon of vinegar added to it. If you pierce them before boiling, they will be have less fat (and calories)!

Tangy Chinese Vegetable Dip

| 1/3 | Cup plum jelly | 1/3 | Cup apple cider vinegar |
| 1/3 | Cup applesauce | 1/2 | Teaspoon brown sugar |

114

Mix well and serve. Double the amount of plum jelly for a more zesty sauce. Also good drizzled over fried noodles.

Salad Dressing

Personalize salad dressings by adding 1/4 cup herb flavored vinegar to commercial mayonnaise, or make oil and vinegar salad dressings with your own herbal vinegars.

Fruit & Vinegar

Wash and mash fresh, well ripened fruit, using 2 cups of vinegar for each cup of fruit. Set in the refrigerator for 4 or 5 days. Strain off the flavored vinegar and heat it to the boiling point. Add 1/2 cup sugar for each cup of vinegar and simmer until the sugar is dissolved. Store in a glass jar. Good fruits for making vinegar are: raspberries, blueberries, blackberries, strawberries and peaches. Combine several fruits for even better flavor. (Lemon and orange go well with most berries.) Plum is an exceptionally good vinegar; drizzle it over a fresh fruit platter for a low calorie taste delight.

Vinegar Marinate

Begin with equal parts white vinegar and water. Add about 3 tablespoons of sugar and a dash of salt for each cup of vinegar. Use this marinate to tenderize both meats and vegetables.

Vinegar & Onions

Wash tiny onions, peel, blanch and cover with a layer of salt. Sit overnight and rinse off the salt. Add enough Vinegar Marinate to cover and boil with spices until the onions are just barely tender (about 10 minutes). For each pound of onions use 1 tablespoon pickling spice, 4 cloves and 4 peppercorns.

Vinegar & Beets

Heat vinegar, water, sugar, and salt (as in Vinegar Marinate) to the boiling point and pour over sliced, fresh cooked or canned beets. Set for at least 24 hours before serving.

Vinegar-Pepper Sauce Supreme

Place an assortment of small whole red and green peppers (or sliced large ones) in a decorative bottle. Use sweet peppers for a mild sauce, hot peppers for a tangy one. Add a couple green onions and a small leek. Fill the jar with vinegar that has been heated to the boiling point. Cap the jar and set aside for at least a month. Use vinegar-pepper sauce on salads (especially pasta salads).

Vinegar-Nut Pie Crust

1/2	Cup butter	1/2	Cup ground nuts
3/4	Cup flour	2	Tablespoons sugar
3/4	Cup oatmeal	1	Tablespoon white vinegar

Melt the butter in a pie pan and then add all the other ingredients. Mix with a fork, then pat the dough into shape. Bake for 15 - 20 minutes at 350°, then fill with fresh fruit and a cornstarch based sauce.

Easiest Vinegar Pie Crust

1 1/3	Cup flour	1	Tablespoon vinegar
1/2	Teaspoon salt	1/3	Cup oil
2	Tablespoons sugar	2	Tablespoons water

Put all ingredients in a pie pan and stir with a fork until the flour is barely moist. Finger press the dough onto the sides and bottom of the pie pan and form a fluted edge along the top. Prick with a fork and bake at 350° until lightly browned. (Or add filling and bake.)

White Vinegar Taffy

2	Cups sugar	1	Teaspoon vanilla extract
1	Tablespoon butter	1/2	Cup water
3	Tablespoons white vinegar		

Combine sugar, vinegar and water and boil to the hard ball stage. Add butter and vanilla and pour onto a greased plate or countertop. When cool enough to touch (but still hot) begin to knead with buttered hands. When the taffy lightens and begins to firm up, cut it into small pieces and wrap in waxed paper to keep it from becoming sticky. Make honey taffy by replacing half of the sugar with honey or butterscotch taffy by replacing half of the sugar with brown sugar and increasing the butter to 2 tablespoons.

A little Vinegar goes a long way-so use the best you can afford.

Teresa's Peanut Butter-Vinegar Fudge

1	Cup chocolate chips	3/4	Cup corn syrup
3 1/2	Cups sugar	1	Tablespoon white vinegar
1/2	Cup butter	3	Cups peanut butter
1 1/2	Cups evaporated milk		
1	Cup marshmallow cream		

In a large saucepan, combine sugar, milk, butter, corn syrup and vinegar. Cook over medium heat, stirring constantly, until mixture comes to a full boil. Boil and stir for 5 minutes, then remove from heat. Add the peanut butter and marshmallow cream and stir until smooth. Pour half of the hot mixture into a bowl with the chocolate chips and stir until smooth. Pour onto a wax paper lined pan and top with the remaining hot mixture. Allow to cool, then cut into squares.

Umeboshi Plums

Make a surprise treat the oriental way. Put a pitted (pickled and salted) umeboshi plum in the middle of a ball made of rice that has been cooked to a sticky consistency.

Mash several umeboshi plums and add enough rice vinegar to form a thick puree. Add a small amount of oil and drizzle over steamed vegetables. Replace the oil with yogurt it makes a good topping for rice cakes.

Vinegar Fish Broth

2	Quarts cold water	1	Cup vinegar
1	Tablespoon salt	2	Small sliced onions
4	Thyme leaves	3	Small cut up carrots

Bring the water to a boil in a large fish kettle. Add the rest of the ingredients and 5 pounds of large pieces of salmon or trout. Simmer gently, until the fish is barely tender. Add a handful of peppercorns and a few sprigs of parsley. All kinds of fish are easier to scale if they are rubbed with vinegar and allowed to set for 5 minutes before scaling.

Best French Dressing

Soak a split clove of garlic for at least 30 minutes in 1 cup of vinegar. Discard the garlic (or add it to soup). Mix in 1 tablespoon each of dry mustard and sugar and 1 teaspoon each of salt and paprika. Add 1 1/2 cups of salad oil and mix well. Use flavored vinegars to vary the taste.

Stuffed Peppers

Stuff large green peppers with cabbage slaw and stack in a stone crock. Cover with vinegar and age 4 weeks before using.

Spiced Mushrooms

1	Pound fresh mushrooms	1	Teaspoon soy sauce
1/2	Cup apple cider vinegar	1	Tablespoon olive oil
1	Teaspoon hot pepper sauce		
1	Tablespoon ginger		
3	Cloves garlic, peeled and chopped.		

Blanch mushrooms in boiling water for 2 minutes, drain and pat dry. Put all ingredients into a jar with a tight lid and refrigerate overnight. Pile mushrooms on spinach leaves and serve with hot garlic toast.

Vinegar Salad

1/2	Cup salad dressing	1/2	Cup vinegar
1	Tablespoon sugar	1	Cup raisins
1/2	Lb. bacon, cooked crisp and crumbled		
1	Cup sunflower kernels		
2	Cups chopped and blanched broccoli		

Half a head of lettuce.

Mix the salad dressing, sugar and vinegar together and drizzle over torn lettuce, raisins, bacon, sunflower kernels and broccoli.

Cherry-Pineapple Vinegar Cake

1	Cup milk	3	Tablespoons vinegar
1	Teaspoon soda	3/4	Lb. flour
3/4	Cup butter	3/4	Cup brown sugar
1	Teaspoon allspice	1/2	Lb. candied cherries
1/2	Lb. candied pineapple		

Stir the vinegar into the milk, add the soda and stir briskly. Cream butter, sugar and flour together and add the fruit and allspice. Fold in the milk and beat well. Bake in a well greased pan at 350° for 1 hour.

Better Boiled Eggs

A splash of vinegar added to the water used to boil eggs will discourage whites from oozing out of cracked eggs.

COOKING TIPS

The most palatable way to take a daily dose of vinegar is to add a small dollop of clover honey to a tablespoon of vinegar and a teaspoon of olive oil. Mix it all together and drip this healthy dressing over a small bowl of greens.

Another way to add calcium to the diet is to crumble feta cheese over torn greens. Use spinach, collards, beet tops, and kale, in addition to lettuce leaves. Sprinkle on a mixture of 2 tablespoons apple cider vinegar, 2 tablespoons honey, and 2 tablespoons water.

Enzymatic browning gives apple cider its color + tang.

Vinegar is used as a bleaching agent on white vegetables. It also prevents enzymatic browning. When foods do not darken in air, they do not develop the off-taste associated with browning. Rice vinegar is also used in salad dressings, marinades, sauces, dips, and spreads.

118

Vinegar acts as a tenderizer on meats and vegetables used in stir-fry dishes.

Vinegar, added to fish dishes, helps to eliminate the traditional fishy odor. It also helps get rid of fish smells at clean up time.

Keep candy and icings smooth and free of gritty sugar granules by adding a few drops of vinegar to the recipe.

A few drops of white vinegar in the water used to boil potatoes will keep them snowy white.

FUN FOR CHILDREN

See Through Eggs
Soak eggs in vinegar for about 24 hours, drain and soak again. In a short time all the egg shells will disappear, leaving clear, wiggly eggs.

Dancing Snowballs
Mix equal parts of water and vinegar and pour it over a handful of mothballs that have been sprinkled with a teaspoon of baking soda. The white 'snowballs' will dance best in a tall vase.

Tangy Citrus Vinegar
Heat three cups of white or champagne vinegar to just under boiling and pour it over a 1 1/2 cups sugar and 1/2 cup of thin cut strips of orange, grapefruit and lemon peel.

Put Vinegar To Work – All Around The Home

*I*n many parts of the country, water for the home comes from underground sources. When this water runs through underground reservoirs it can dissolve minerals out of rock formations. Limestone, which is mostly calcium carbonate, dissolves especially easily.

This hard water carries the dissolved limestone until it finds an object to deposit it on. The inside of plumbing pipes, bathroom and kitchen fixtures, shower walls and curtains and washer lint traps encourage minerals to precipitate out of water. These minerals show up as a rock-hard coating which can be difficult to clean without scratching metal surfaces. In a short time these hard water minerals build up into a dirty looking, flaky white scale on bathroom and kitchen surfaces. This is the same stuff that produces stalagmites and stalactites in limestone caves. It can be just as hard as these natural wonders, but it is not nearly as pretty! Fortunately, vinegar dissolves calcium carbonate, as well as scale from other minerals.

HOW TO CHOOSE A VINEGAR

Most cleaning and laundry chores call for white vinegar. It has a mild odor and does not have anything in it to leave a stain on fabrics. Apple cider vinegar is a good choice for cleaning that calls for giving the air a pleasant, apple-fresh scent. Either one leaves a room smelling as if it has just been cleaned.

Throughout this chapter, whenever a cleaning tip does not specify the kind of vinegar to be used, white vinegar is usually the best one to use. But, it is always possible to do the cleaning chore with any kind of vinegar. The choice is always yours!

WHEN TO CLEAN WITH VINEGAR

Vinegar is the cleaner of choice for those with allergies, asthma or a sensitivity to harsh chemicals. It also appeals to those who are interested in protecting the environment from pollution, and is the cleaning product of choice for the thrifty consumer.

Vinegar's acid character makes it especially useful for neutralizing the effect of alkaline-based cleaning products. This includes most soaps and detergents. Vinegar also has the ability to dissolve the dulling film these products can leave behind.

Copper (and compounds that contain copper) can be cleaned with vinegar. When metal develops a green tarnish it usually means there is copper in it. This green coating can be seen on objects that are 100% copper, as well as on copper compounds such as brass and bronze. Brass can develop a dull, greenish discoloration because it is mostly copper, with some zinc mixed into it. Bronze also has a copper base. The copper in bronze is mixed with tin (and sometimes a bit of zinc, too).

Copper tarnish is poisonous.

WHEN NOT TO CLEAN WITH VINEGAR

Just as important as when to use vinegar, is when not to use it. Vinegar will tarnish silver, so never expose it to vinegar, unless you want it to instantly look old and dirty. And, never, ever soak pearls in vinegar, as it will dissolve them! Also use caution around jewelry made of opal, coral or ivory.

If you reuse plastic bags, such as bread wrappers, never turn the bag inside-out, so that a food with vinegar in it touches the colored ink of the bag label design. Labels may contain coloring dyes that release lead into food when soaked in vinegar.

IN THE KITCHEN

Grandmother knew the value of vinegar in the kitchen, and she used it for more than cooking! All sorts of viruses, bacteria and fungus can grow on kitchen surfaces. Keeping everything clean and dry helps to eliminate them and the sickness they can bring. Vinegar

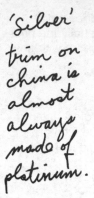

'Silver' trim on china is almost always made of platinum.

can be a big help in doing this. Use white vinegar for its antibiotic and antiseptic qualities, or use apple cider vinegar to add the fresh aroma of ripe fall apples to vinegar's power. For a very special effect, clean with your own homemade herbal vinegar. Herbal vinegar can add a very special aroma to your kitchen, giving guests a hint of the foods you prepare. When scientific research looks at old-time home remedies, they have often been surprised to find many really work! Grandmother may not have been able to explain chemical reactions, but she knew her remedies worked.

Miscellaneous Glassware

To clean dull glassware, immerse pieces in a container filled with white vinegar. Let soak for 30 minutes, then scrub with a soft brush dipped in warm, sudsy water. Rinse in clear water, then rinse again in a sink full of very warm water with 1/2 cup white vinegar added to it. Dry with a soft cloth and see how your glassware sparkles!

Lead Crystal

Fine crystal should always be washed and dried by hand. A bit of white vinegar in the rinse water will help keep them from developing a scummy buildup of dulling minerals. To wash: place a rubber mat (or a dish towel) in the bottom of the sink. Add enough hot water and detergent to make enough nice sudsy water to allow you to completely submerge each piece. Wash thoroughly and rinse in hot water with several tablespoons of white vinegar added to it. Dry with a very absorbent cotton towel.

Fine China

When hand washing good dishes, a splash of white vinegar in the last rinse will help prevent streaks and spots - but only use it on china that does not have gold or silver trim. Vinegar can cause metal trims on china to discolor. After drying plates, slip an inexpensive paper plate between each piece of china and you will reduce the chance of dishes being chipped.

Ceramic Dishes, Bowls & Casseroles

Clean encrusted foods from ceramic cookware by scouring them with a nylon scrubber dipped in white vinegar.

Vase Cleaning

Small vases often have tiny openings that make cleaning difficult. Use a small brush dipped in full strength white vinegar to scrub them clean.

Better Vase Cleaning

If you do not have exactly the right size brush for scrubbing the inside of a small vase, use vinegar, water and rice to scour it. Put a handful of rice in the vase and fill it 1/3 of the way full with a half and half mixture of white vinegar and cold water. Shake well, let set for 30 seconds, shake again. Empty out the rice and liquid, rinse in water and vinegar, and set the vase upside down to dry.

Even Better Vase Cleaning

For really tough cleaning jobs, put a few tablespoons of fine sand in a dirty vase. Fill to 1/3 full with a mixture of half white vinegar and half hot water. Shake until deposits are removed, empty and rinse well before drying.

Appliance Cords

Keep electric cords, especially white ones, clean and free of food smears by wiping them frequently with a cloth dampened with white vinegar. (Always unplug electric cords before cleaning them!)

Small Appliances

Can openers, toasters, mixers, blenders and such can be wiped down with a cloth wrung out of white vinegar, then buffed dry. They will stay nice looking longer, and work better, if kept clean. Always spray vinegar on a cloth (or use a cloth wrung out of vinegar); never spray the appliance directly. Liquid could enter the air vents over motors and damage internal parts. (ALWAYS unplug appliances before cleaning.)

Blender Buttons

White vinegar, on a cotton swab, does a good job of cleaning push buttons and control knobs on blenders and food processors. Rub the vinegar into the small spaces around and between buttons, too.

Mixers

One of the hardest cleaning jobs in the kitchen is getting food splashes off of the underside of mixers. Make this chore easier by wrapping a vinegar dampened cloth around the mixer for a few minutes. Wipe off loose dirt; repeat if necessary.

Can Opener Cleaning

Can opener blades often harbor dried-on food and bits of unidentified gunk, in even the most spotless of kitchens. Soak removable blades in white vinegar until the encrusted food is soft enough to scrub off. Use a vinegar dampened cotton swab to clean the air vents over the motor, being careful not to push dried food into the motor housing.

Really Dirty Refrigerators

The top of tall appliances such as refrigerators and some freezers can collect a layer of gummy dirt. Dust settles up there, gets mixed with grease in the air and then steam from cooking cements it together into a cleaning challenge. Vacuum as much of the gunk up as possible. Then spray a damp sponge with full strength vinegar and drizzle liquid for hand washing dishes over the vinegar. Pat the sponge over the entire refrigerator top and let it soak for 15 minutes. Use the sponge to wipe the stuck-on dirt off. (It will come off easily now.) Rinse with a solution of hot water and a dash of white vinegar, then buff dry. A light coating of wax or polish on the top of the refrigerator will help to keep greasy dust from sticking to it.

Gas Stove Grates

Boil iron burner grates from gas stoves, for about 10 minutes, in water with a cup of vinegar added to it. They will be much easier to clean.

Stove Tops

Wipe spatters and grease from stovetops with a cloth wrung out of a solution made from 1/2 cup white vinegar, 1/2 cup water, and 1 teaspoon liquid detergent.

Oven Cleaner

Put 3 cups of water into a shallow baking dish and heat oven to 300°. Turn the oven off and let set for 20 minutes. Replace the water with 2 cups of ammonia and allow to set overnight. To 1/2 cup of the ammonia, add 1/2 cup white vinegar and 2 cups baking soda. Smooth this mixture over oven surfaces and allow to set for 20 minutes. Wipe away the cleaner and rinse with clear water.

Oven Racks

Spray oven racks with vinegar and let set until they dry naturally. Then place them in a tub of very hot water with 1 cup of vinegar and a tablespoon of dishwasher detergent added to it. Let the racks soak until the water has cooled. Repeat soaking process and then wipe the racks down with a sponge.

Dishwashers

Dishwashers, especially those used in hard water areas, often attract an unsightly buildup of lime and other minerals. In addition to discoloring the inside of the dishwasher, minerals can damage its working parts. Running the dishwasher for a complete washing cycle, with no detergent in it, can dissolve these deposits. Instead, put 2 cups white vinegar in the bottom of the dishwasher. Stop the machine before the drying cycle begins and wipe the top and sides down with a soft cloth. Never dry the bottom of the dishwasher, as many brands rely on a small amount of water remaining in the bottom to protect seals from drying out and being ruined.

Quick Kitchen Deodorizing Treatment

Dampen a sponge or cloth with full strength apple cider vinegar and place it over a heat or air conditioning register. Allow air to circulate through the vinegar-wet cloth for 15 to 20 minutes and the air will smell fresh and pure.

Emily's Favorite Kitchen Deodorizer

Keep a small pump spray bottle of water, with 2 tablespoons of white vinegar added to it, handy in the kitchen. Whenever odor is a problem, a few puffs into the air will neutralize it. An old pump hair spray bottle works well, because it puts out a fine, easily diffused mist. Use when cooking fish, cabbage, after boil overs or anytime the air needs a quick freshening. Or, simmer 1/4 cup vinegar in a pot of water, uncovered, to clear the air of lingering cooking odors. Add 1/2 teaspoon of cinnamon to the water for an extra special air cleaner. Or, simmer 1/4 cup vinegar in a pot of water, uncovered, to clear the air of lingering cooking odors. Add 1/2 teaspoon of cinnamon to the water for an extra special air cleaner.

Coffee Pots

Coffee oils are very thick and sticky, so they tend to collect on the inside of pots and on percolator parts. When they become old, these oils decompose and release the acids that give coffee a sour taste and rancid smell. An occasional touch of vinegar will dissolve coffee oils and so keep coffee pots from developing rancid odors. Just add 1 tablespoon of vinegar to a full pot of hot water and let it set for 10 minutes. Rinse well and the pot will make excellent coffee again. For very corroded pots, use half water, half white vinegar.

Microwave Cleaning Magic

Soften cooked-on food particles by placing a heat safe bowl containing 1/2 cup water and 1/2 cup vinegar in the oven. Heat until the solution begins to boil, then run the microwave, on its highest setting, for an additional 30 seconds. Spills and caked-on foods will wipe off with ease.

Microwave Odor Remover

Place a cup of water with 2 tablespoons of apple cider vinegar in it in the microwave. Bring the mixture to a boil and then let it set for 3 minutes. The oven will smell fresh and clean again. This is especially good for removing fish or popcorn odors.

Electric Knives

Wipe all surfaces with a cloth wrung out of a solution of sudsy water and vinegar. Give special attention to crevices around blade mounting areas. Finish by wiping the electric cord and wall plug.

Teapots need cleaned, too !

Enamel Ware

Bleach stains from enamel cookware by boiling a few cups of white vinegar in them.

Thermos Cleaner

Fill a stained vacuum bottle with a mixture made of 2 parts white vinegar to 1 part cold water. Let stand for an hour, then add a tablespoon of uncooked rice and shake for several minutes. Rinse several times and wipe dry.

Kitchen Counter Tops

To preserve glossy surfaces, use vinegar and water to wipe down lightly soiled counter tops. Use detergent, soap or ammonia based products only when really needed, as they break down wax-based polishes. Laminated plastic counter tops (such as Formica®) need to be kept covered with a layer of wax to protect them from tiny cuts and scratches that will eventually make the surface look dull.

Clean AND disinfect.

Counter Top Scrubber

Make a great, disposable, counter top scrubber by dipping a piece of old nylon hose in vinegar and using it to scrub globs of stuck-on goo off laminated plastic counter tops. This combination has enough cleaning power to remove the mess, yet will not scratch the surface. (Really hard globs can be allowed to soak for a few minutes.)

Very Dirty Counter Tops

When counter tops have really hard globs of foods or other materials on them, use a vinegar compress to loosen the dirt. Soaking the material loose will save the work of scrubbing and scraping and, more importantly, save wear and tear on the counter top.

Crumb Catcher

A cloth dampened with a light spray of vinegar will catch a whole counter top of crumbs, without spreading them all over. While you are chasing crumbs, do not forget the crumb catcher in the toaster!

Drain Cleaner

Slow-running drains can often be improved by treating them with baking soda and vinegar. Begin by sprinkling 1/4 cup soda into the drain. Immediately pour 1/2 cup vinegar into the drain. Allow it to foam and sizzle for a few minutes. When the action has stopped, pour at least 2 quarts of boiling water down the drain.

Drain & Septic Treatment

Plumbing lines that empty into septic systems can benefit from an occasional bacteria boosting treatment. Begin by using a vinegar and baking soda drain cleaner (see above) in all drains. When the drains are clean and free-running, pour 1 package dry yeast and 2/3 cup brown sugar into the toilet and flush twice. Do this about once a month and the system will work efficiently for years.

Drain Deodorizer

Pour 1/2 cup vinegar down each drain, every week. The vinegar will keep the drains smelling sweet (and discourage clogs, too)!

Magic Garbage Disposer Freshener

Mix equal parts apple cider vinegar and water and freeze the mixture in an ice cube tray. Store the frozen cubes in a plastic bag. Then, grind a few of these special freshener cubes in the disposer each week for instant cleaning that will also leave it smelling fresh.

Vinegar Magic For Aluminum Pots and Pans

Aluminum pans become discolored if they get a lot of exposure to salty foods, ammonia or cleaning products that contain ammonia. If 1/2 cup white vinegar, with a couple of cups of water added to it, is occasionally boiled in such pans, staining will be kept to a minimum. For lightly stained cookware; make a paste of white vinegar and baking soda. Spread over stained aluminum cooking utensils. Remove with fine superfine steel wool.

For medium stains: mix the baking soda with an equal amount of cream of tartar, then stir in the vinegar. For badly stained pans: use baking soda and cream of tartar (as for medium stains) and mix with vinegar which has been mixed half and half with liquid detergent.

Copper Pans

When copper pans oxidize, a green film forms. This is called verdigris and, while it is a bit unsightly on the outside of pans, it helps them do a better job of absorbing heat.

Iron forms rust, copper forms verdigris.

Green oxide on the inside of pans this is a bigger problem - it is poisonous. This is why most pans only use copper on the outside, or sandwiched between two other metals. If a copper pan develops these patches of green on the inside, seriously consider throwing it away. To clean verdigris from the inside of copper pans: fill with water, add 1/3 cup vinegar and 1/3 cup salt.

Boil for 10 minutes and scrub vigorously. Rinse well.

Copper Cleaner
1	cup white vinegar	1/4 cup flour
1/2	cup water	1/2 cup salt
1/2	cup powdered detergent	

Whisk all ingredients together, then slowly heat in a double boiler until the detergent is dissolved and the mixture begins to thicken. Set aside until cool. To use, wipe onto copper with a small cloth, let set for 30 seconds, then wipe off with a clean cloth.

Copper & Brass
Brass and copper will sparkle and tarnish will melt away if wiped down with 2 tablespoons catsup and 1 tablespoon vinegar. Polish until completely dry with a clean cloth.

Quick Copper & Glass Cleaner
Make a brass and copper cleaner by combining equal parts of lemon juice and vinegar. Wipe it on with a paper towel, then polish with a dry towel and discard.

Teflon + Silver-Stone are brand names for no-stick cookware.

No-Stick Pans
Mineral salts from hard water can build up on the surfaces of pans coated with fluorocarbon compounds. These no-stick coatings should not be scrubbed with harsh chemicals or steel wool pads. Whitish mineral stains can be removed by boiling 2 cups of water and 1/3 cup white vinegar in the pan for a few minutes, then wipe the pan dry with a soft cloth.

Foil & Vinegar Scrubbers
Make your own scrubber for removing cooked on food from pans and baking dishes. Simply crumple up a wad of aluminum foil (new or used), dip it in vinegar and rub the cooked on food away. Extra hard spots can be soaked in vinegar for a few minutes before scrubbing.

Vinegar & Apple Cleaner
Remove stains from the inside of aluminum cookware by boiling 1 quart of water, 1/2 cup white vinegar and 1 cup apple peels for 15 minutes.

Rust Stains From Metal
Rust stains on stainless steel sinks can be wiped away by scouring with salt, dampened with vinegar.

Plastic Food Containers

Plastic storage containers pick up and hold food odors very easily. Keep them odor-free by soaking them in sudsy warm water, with a generous splash of white vinegar added to it.

Refrigerator and Freezer Gaskets

Wipe the gaskets around refrigerator and freezer doors with a mild detergent solution to keep them free of dirt and grease. If mold begins to form on the gaskets, remove it with white vinegar, then rinse with clear water before drying.

Spotless Glassware

A splash of vinegar added to rinse water will keep glasses from water spotting. It kills germs, too.

Iron Pots

Use vinegar and hay to revitalize iron pans that have rust spots. Fill the pot with hay, add 1/4 cup vinegar and enough water to cover the hay. Boil for 1 hour and wipe the rust away.
Rhubarb may be substituted for the hay.

Clean like grandma, use vinegar

Cabbage Cleaner

Pewter cleans up easily if rubbed with cabbage leaves. Just wet the leaves in vinegar and dip them in salt before using them to buff the pewter. Be sure to rinse with cool water and dry thoroughly.

Pewter Paste

Clean pewter with a paste made of 1 tablespoon salt, 1 tablespoon flour, and enough vinegar to just barely make the mixture wet. Smear it on discolored pewter and allow to dry. Rub or brush the dried paste off, rinse in hot water, and buff dry.

Grease Free Dish Washing

A half cup vinegar added to dish washing water cuts grease and lets you use less soap.

Stuck-On Food

Soak or simmer stuck-on food in 2 cups of water and 1/2 cup of vinegar. The food will soften and lift off in a few minutes.

Self-Defrosting Refrigerators

The water collecting tray under self-defrosting refrigerators and freezers should be washed occasionally in soapy water. Any buildup of minerals can be dissolved by soaking in white vinegar. A teaspoon or two of vinegar in the tray will retard the growth of bacteria and help prevent moldy smells.

Sanitize Cutting Boards

Disinfect wood cutting boards at least once a week (and after each time they are used to cut meat) by applying a liberal coating of salt. Let the salt set for 5 minutes, then wash with 1/2 cup vinegar. This keeps cutting boards sweet-smelling and sanitary. Traditional wood boards should be wiped down with vegetable oil once in a while, too. Another way to clean, disinfect and deodorize wood cutting blocks is to rub them with baking soda, then spray on full strength vinegar. Let sit for 5 minutes, then rinse in clear water. It will bubble and froth as these two natural chemicals interact.

BATHROOMS

Bathrooms are always a special cleaning challenge. They sprout mildew and mold, attract odors and breed tub and shower slime. Tradition says the North African general, Hannibal, used the fact that vinegar weakens rock in his march through the Alps from Spain to Italy. You may not have an immediate need to relocate a boulder so your elephants can cross a mountain range, but you may went to try some of these ways to ease cleaning chores:

Shower Heads

When heavy mineral deposits are visible on the shower head, it usually means these salts have been deposited inside, too. Unscrew the fixture and soak it in full strength white vinegar. The vinegar will dissolve and soften the buildup. If the small openings are clogged, use a toothpick or small nail to remove the minerals that have been deposited on them. Then scrub with an old toothbrush and rinse well. Keep shower heads sparkling bright by wiping them down once a week with white vinegar. Give the tiny nozzle openings special attention, so that mineral precipitations do not develop. A thin coating of wax can help prevent hard water deposits from sticking to the metal.

Shower Curtains

A shower curtain that is stained with mildew or mold can be revived by soaking it in a laundry tub of warm water with 2 cups of white vinegar added to it. Let it soak for a couple of hours (or over night) and then wash in warm, sudsy water and dry in the sun. Wipe down the shower curtain on a regular basis with white vinegar and it will be less likely to develop mildew or mold stains. Just spray the bottom fourth of the curtain with white vinegar and wipe it off with a soft cloth.

Keep It Shiny

After wiping chrome, brass or other metal bathroom fixtures with vinegar and water, dry completely and apply two light coats of wax. They will look bright and shiny longer, clean up easier next time, and will resist the buildup of hard water mineral salts.

Ceramic Tile

Floors, back splashes, shower walls and such will shine their best if rinsed in a mild vinegar and water solution, then buffed dry. Keep ceramic tile showers free of soap scum and hard water salts buildup by drying after each use. A synthetic chamois cloth does a wonderful job of wiping down tile because it absorbs water so well. Keep the cloth fresh and clean by washing it occasionally in a mild liquid detergent, then rinsing it in vinegar to neutralize the soap and minerals it will be constantly wiping up.

Hair Rollers, Brushes & Combs

Over time, hair rollers, brushes and combs can pick up coatings of hair spray, mousse and setting gels. This buildup attracts dirt and dust, turning it a dark and sticky. Remove this coating by soaking rollers, brushes and combs for an hour in a quart of warm water with a cup of white vinegar added to it. Then scrub with an old toothbrush that has been dipped in liquid detergent. The buildup will now come off easily. Follow with a clear water rinse, then a rinse in warm water with a dash of white vinegar. Blot most of the water off and air dry, in the sun if possible.

Plastic Wall Tile

Plastic tile scratches easily and attracts hard water mineral buildup. Clean it with non-abrasive white vinegar and protect it with a light wax.

Soap Film Remover

Shower walls, in particular, seem to attract scummy soap film. Vinegar and baking soda can eat right through it! Simply take 1 cup baking soda and add enough white vinegar to make a thick, frothy cream. Spread it over areas where soap film has built up and let set for 5 minutes. Wipe off with a soft brush or sponge, rinse in water with some white vinegar added to it and buff dry.

Extra Power Soap Film Treatment

Mix together 1/4 cup white vinegar and 1/4 cup ammonia. Add enough baking soda to make a thick paste. Spread this mixture over the area that has a coating of soap film. Let set for 10 minutes, then remove with a medium-bristled brush. Follow with a rinse of cool water, with a little vinegar added to it.

Use ammonia with care.

Soap Film Preventive

Prevent soap film buildup by rinsing all exposed surfaces, every week, with a solution of vinegar and water. A cup of white vinegar to a quart of water is about right for hard water areas, a cup to a gallon of water for soft water areas.

Bathroom Odors

Instead of using an aerosol air freshener to fight bathroom odors, keep a pump spray bottle of vinegar water handy. Just fill the bottle with water and 1 tablespoon white vinegar. Whenever odor relief is needed, a few sprays will release a fine mist to neutralize odors. For best results, use a pump sprayer of the type hair spray comes in. It will release a very fine mist, spreading the vinegar into the air rapidly. A mist with vinegar in it, instead of a floral scent, is especially good for households where someone has hay fever or is allergic to flowers and grasses. Vinegar neutralizes odors without adding a fragrance that can trigger allergies and add to indoor pollution.

Hair In The Sink

Cleaning pesky hair clippings from the sink can be a messy, frustrating job. Make it easy with a dash of vinegar. Simply spray vinegar on a piece of bathroom tissue and use it to wipe out the sink. Fold the tissue over the hair, wipe again and discard the tissue and hair.

Better Wet Wipes

Mix 1 cup vinegar, 1 cup water and 1 tablespoon liquid detergent in a bowl. Wet small pieces of clean, soft cloth in the vinegar mixture, then wring them out. Place the cloths in a tightly capped container. Use wet wipes for cleaning and moving spots on faucets and fixture handles, drains, around tub enclosures and sinks, and even on the outside surfaces of toilets. They also do a good job cleaning windows, walls and floors. Make disposable wet wipes by substituting sheets of extra heavy paper towels for pieces of cloth. They are great for wiping up unpleasant bathroom messes. Splatters, spots and isolated fingerprints on windows and mirrors can also be removed by wiping them down with vinegar wet wipes.

VINEGAR ACTS AGAINST GERMS

Vinegar contains a host of germ fighting components. It is has both antibiotic and antiseptic properties. Vinegar not only can kill bacteria, its presence slows future growth. One of the best things about cleaning with vinegar is its action on mold and mildew. Mold and mildew are not dirt. They are living, plantlike growths. That means cleaning the part that shows is not enough to get rid of them. These fungus growths have to be killed, all the way to their roots, or they will immediately grow back.

And that is why vinegar is such a good cleaning product. It

has the ability to actually kill mold and mildew spores that cause new growth. Vinegar is a completely biodegradable product. Nature can easily break it down into components that feed and nurture plant life. This makes it superior to chemical cleaners that poison the soil today and can remain in it and destroy plant life for many years.

Dryrot + corn smut are also fungus.

Mildew

That slimy growth in showers, around tubs and in other damp places is really a plant. It is a soft, spongy fungus that can be white as well as black or purplish in color. Mildew grows best where it is dark and the air is warm and wet and stagnant. It thrives in showers and tubs, where it lives on body oil, dirt particles and soap scum.

Vinegar helps to remove the dirt, oil and soap that provide its food. It also leaves behind an acid environment to slow the future growth of mildew. So, the cure for any area attacked by mildew, mold or other fungus is to keep it dry, give it lots of sunshine and regularly rinse it with a strong vinegar solution!

Mildew And Mold Removal

The metal edges of shower and tub surrounds are especially attractive to mold and mildew. Scrub them down with a piece of crumbled up foil that has been dipped in full strength vinegar. Use a toothbrush dipped in vinegar for crevices and corners. Rinse with clear water, then with water and vinegar and buff dry. Use white vinegar to dissolve soap film and kill mold and mildew. It will leave the bathroom smelling fresh and clean. Use apple cider vinegar for the same cleaning power, but with a stronger, fresher, longer lasting fragrance.

Vinegar enhances the power of other cleaning substances.

Many folk recipes combine vinegar with other household supplies for safe cleaning and disinfecting. Chemical cleaners use synthetic chemicals that are not always as environmentally safe as more natural, organic compounds. Among the more popular substances which have traditionally been used in combination with vinegar are baking soda, borax, chalk, pumice, oil, salt, washing soda, and wax. To vinegar, add:

- Baking soda to absorb odors, deodorize and as a mild abrasive.
- Borax to disinfect, deodorize, and stop the growth of mold.
- Chalk for a mild, non abrasive cleaner.

- Oil to preserve and shine.
- Pumice to remove stains or polish surfaces.
- Salt for a mild abrasive.
- Washing soda to cut heavy grease.
- Wax to protect and shine.

DO NOT SEAL A FOAMING VINEGAR
MIXTURE IN A TIGHTLY CAPPED CONTAINER!

PLEASE NOTE: Some ingredients, when added to a vinegar solution, will produce a frothy foam. This is a natural chemical reaction and is not dangerous in an open container.

Cleaners you make yourself cost pennies, instead of the dollars super market cleaners cost. And, what is much more significant, the compounds you put together are safe, natural, and easy on the environment. Commercial equivalents cost more and may be more damaging to the environment. Using vinegar to clean and disinfect is more than the inexpensive choice from a simpler time. It is the natural choice!

A collection of useful formulas for cleaning and polishing with vinegar based solutions follow. As with all cleaning products, test these old-time solutions to cleaning problems before using them. Always try them out on an inconspicuous area of rugs, upholstery, or clothing.

Fresh Air
Make your own kind-to-the-environment air freshener. Put the following into a pump spray bottle: 1 teaspoon baking soda, 1 tablespoon vinegar, and 2 cups of water. After the foaming stops, put on the lid and shake well. Spray this mixture into the air for instant freshness.

Water Resistant Furniture Polish
An excellent furniture polish can be made from vinegar and lemon oil. Use 3 parts vinegar to 1 part oil for a light weight polish. (Use 1 part vinegar to 3 parts oil for a heavy duty polish.) An oil and vinegar combination works well for cleaning and polishing. This is because vinegar dissolves and brings up dirt and oil enriches the wood.

Dusting
Dusting will go much faster if your dust cloth is dampened with a mixture made of half vinegar and half olive oil. When the vinegar evaporates, the wood is left clean, beautiful and it will have a mild fragrance.

Appliances

Appliances sparkle if cleaned with a vinegar and borax cleaner. Mix 1 teaspoon borax, 1/4 cup vinegar, and 2 cups hot water and put it into a spray bottle. Spray it on greasy smears and wipe off with a cloth or sponge.

Shiny Countertops

Counter tops will shine if wiped down with a mixture of 1 teaspoon liquid soap, 3 tablespoons vinegar, 1/2 teaspoon oil, and 1/2 cup water.

Toilet Cleaner

An excellent toilet cleaner can be made from 1 cup borax and 1 cup vinegar. Pour the vinegar all over the stained area of the toilet; then sprinkle the borax over the vinegar. Allow it all to soak for 2 hours. Then simply brush and flush.

Painted Surfaces

Shine and clean painted surfaces with 1 tablespoon cornstarch, 1/4 cup vinegar, and 2 cups hot water. Spray it on and wipe the paint dry immediately. Rub until it shines.

Leather Shoes

Preserve leather shoes and remove dirt by rubbing them with a vinegar based cleaner. Mix together 1 tablespoon vinegar, 1 tablespoon alcohol, 1 teaspoon vegetable oil and 1/2 teaspoon liquid soap. Wipe it on, then brush until the shoes gleam.

Shower Doors

Water scale build up on glass shower doors can be removed with alum and vinegar. Dissolve 1 teaspoon alum in 1/4 cup vinegar. Wipe it on the glass and scrub with a soft brush. Rinse with lots of water and buff until completely dry. (Alum is aluminum sulfate.)

Vinyl Furniture

Soft vinyl surfaces are best cleaned with 1/2 cup vinegar, 2 teaspoons liquid soap, and 1/2 cup water. Use a soft cloth to wipe this mixture onto vinyl furniture, then rinse with clear water and wipe dry.

Carpet Stains

Remove light carpet stains with a paste made of salt and vinegar. Dissolve 2 tablespoons salt in 1/2 cup vinegar. Rub this into carpet stains, let it dry and vacuum up the residue. Remove heavy carpet stains with a paste made of salt, borax, and vinegar. Dissolve 2 tablespoons salt and 2 tablespoons borax in 1/2 cup vinegar. Rub this into carpet stains, let it dry and vacuum.

Carpet Cleaner
1 cup white vinegar
1/4 cup rubbing alcohol
1 teaspoon liquid detergent
Mix well, then pat gently onto soiled spots. Blot off and rinse with clear water. Repeat as necessary.

Easy Highchair Cleaning
Wash baby's highchair quickly and easily in the shower. Simply set the chair in the shower, spray with full strength white vinegar and let set for 3 minutes. Then turn the shower on for another 3 minutes. A quick buffing with a brush will now loosen any dried on food and another quick rinse will complete the job. The chair will be shiny clean, with no hard scrubbing or scraping and no dangerous chemical residue will remain that could be a danger to the baby.

Baby Odors
Save on utilities, neutralize odors, humidify and safety-proof baby's room with one simple trick! Take a damp towel, direct from the washing machine, and spray it with white vinegar. Hang the towel over the top of the door to baby's room. As the towel dries it will control odors, add moisture to the air and prevent the door from closing all the way, so the little one cannot accidentally lock his or herself in the room.

Sanitizing Toys
Wipe down plastic dolls, blocks, cars and other toys with a cloth wrung out of a solution made of 1 part vinegar and 4 parts water. Or, spray full strength white vinegar onto a damp cloth and use it to wipe dirt and germs from toys.

HOW TO CLEAN WITH VINEGAR

Vinegar is a cost efficient cleaner, so be generous with it. In general, begin cleaning by removing loose dirt with a sweeper, brush, dust cloth, or just shake it off. Then scrape or peel off any lumps or globs of dirt. Remove what remains with detergent, water and white vinegar.

For best results, keep your cleaning equipment clean. The best cleaning machine in the house is usually that old toothbrush that reaches all the places nothing else will. Rinse it out once in a while in full strength vinegar, shake it partly dry, and then allow it to dry in the sun.

Bedrooms are a haven for dust balls, stale air and musty smelling closets. Offices present their own problems with assorted chemical stains and paper bits. Vinegar can help solve all these problems.

Gentle All-Purpose Cleaner

Fill a spray bottle almost full of water, then add 1/4 cup white vinegar and 3 tablespoons liquid detergent (the kind used to wash dishes by hand). Use a few squirts of this gentle preparation to clean away light dust and dirt before moisture in the air turns them into a sticky film that is more difficult to remove. Use this gentle all-purpose cleaner on chair railings, window frames, baseboards and anywhere else dust or dirt tends to accumulate.

Glass or Plastic Beads

Dip strands of beads used as curtains or room dividers in a quart of warm water to which 1 teaspoon liquid detergent has been mixed. Rinse in another quart of water to which 1 tablespoon white vinegar has been added. Blot dry with a towel, then finish drying with a hair dryer, set to low heat.

One-Pass Sweeping

A broom will pick up more dust if it is sprayed with vinegar water. Just put a cup of warm water in a pump spray bottle and add 1 cup vinegar. Spray the broom before using, and occasionally during use.

Louvered Doors and Shutters

Remove dirt, dust and musty odors from louvered surfaces with vinegar and a paint stirring stick (available, free, at most paint stores). Simply wrap a soft cloth over the end of the flat stick, spray it with vinegar, then run it over and under each louver.

Revitalize and Deodorize Drapes

Remove musty or smoky odors from drapes — and take out fine wrinkles at the same time! Mix 1 tablespoon white vinegar with 2 cups warm water and place the mixture in a pump spray bottle. Set to 'fine mist' and spritz each drapery panel lightly, without removing the drapes from the windows. As they dry, most wrinkles will disappear, along with stale odors.

Caution: Always spot test fabrics before using ANY chemical (even water) on them.

Fiberglass Drapes

Fiberglass is, in many ways, a wonderful material. But when it comes time to wash drapes, fiberglass requires great care. These drapes must never be washed in the washing machine or put in the dryer! The agitation of the washer and the tumbling of the dryer, will break, crack and pulverize the glass fibers. Not only will washing machines and dryers weaken (and eventually destroy) the drapes, tiny fiberglass particles will be deposited in the appliances. These little pieces of glass will cause great itching and irritation for anyone who wears clothes exposed to them!

Wash fiberglass drapes by hanging them on a clothes line and spraying them, gently, with a hose. Follow with a spray of vinegar and water from a pump spray bottle (1 tablespoon of vinegar to each 2 cups of water). This will keep them smelling fresh and clean. If it is inconvenient to hang fiberglass drapes outside, they may be dipped in a laundry tub of sudsy water, rinsed in clear water, then dipped in a mild vinegar and water solution. Remember to THOROUGHLY rinse out the laundry tub after washing fiberglass drapes!

Air Freshener
Pure white vinegar makes a great freshener for stale air. Simply use a pump spray to deliver a fine mist to musty areas or to remove cooking and smoking odors. Use white vinegar for a clear, unscented freshener and use apple cider vinegar for a longer lasting freshener.

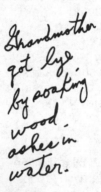

Grandmother got lye by soaking wood ashes in water.

Fireplace Ashes
A vinegar spray can keep fireplace ashes from flying all over the house during fireplace cleaning. Simply spray the ashes with vinegar and water before beginning (1 tablespoon vinegar to 2 cups water). Shovel the ashes onto newspapers that have also been dampened with a spray of water and vinegar. Continue to spray the ashes frequently and flying dust particles will be prevented. Putting vinegar on the ashes also helps to neutralize this strong alkali. Prevent alkali burns on your hands by rinsing them in water and vinegar as soon as the job is finished. Rinse all of the tools you use for this job in a strong solution of vinegar and water, too.

Brighten Lights
Get the most from your lighting dollars by keeping light bulbs clean and free of dust and dirt. Wipe cool bulbs with a cloth dampened in vinegar water (1 tablespoon vinegar to a quart of water). Always clean bulbs with current turned OFF!

Light fixtures, chimneys, reflectors, and diffusers also need to be cleaned regularly. Dip them in sudsy water, then rinse in water with some white vinegar added to it. As with light bulbs, always clean AFTER they have completely cooled! Use a mild vinegar and water solution for plastic parts, a strong one for glass items.

Ballpoint Ink

Pen marks on painted walls and woodwork can usually be lifted by soaking them in white vinegar. Dribble full strength vinegar on marks and allow soaking for 10 to 15 minutes.

Walls

Wash painted walls with a gentle detergent and then rinse them in warm water and white vinegar.

Ceilings

Lightly soiled ceilings can be washed and rinsed in one operation. To half a bucket of water, add 1 tablespoon liquid dish detergent and 1/2 cup white vinegar. Wipe a 3 foot square of ceiling clean, then dry with a soft cloth to prevent streaking.

Glass and Ceramic Candlesticks

Soak glass and ceramic candlesticks in very warm water with plenty of detergent in it. Wipe wax residue off with a soft cloth or sponge. Then, rinse in hot water with a bit of white vinegar in it. Put a coating of oil in the candle-holding well to make it easier to remove old candles.

Lamp Shades

Before throwing a hopelessly stained or misshapen lamp shade away, you might want to give it a chance to redeem itself. Make a sudsy solution of white vinegar, liquid detergent, and lukewarm water in a laundry tub. Immerse the end of the shade with the heaviest soil buildup first. Swish it around a little, then turn the lamp shade over, with the opposite end sub-merged in the water. Turn the shade over and repeat the process. Swish it around again and drain the water out of the laundry tub. Fill the tub with cool water, add 1 cup white vinegar, and rinse the shade thoroughly. Blot most of the water from the lamp shade and finish drying out of the sun, and without heat.

Mildewy Windows

Windows that are frequently damp often grow mildew and mold in their corners and on their frames. Use full strength white vinegar to remove all traces of mildew and mold. Any spores that are missed will encourage rapid regrowth.

Good Window Cleaner

1 Tablespoon vinegar	2	Drops liquid detergent
1 Tablespoon ammonia	1	Cup water

Mix all ingredients together and store in a pump spray bottle. Spray onto windows and wipe off with wadded up newspaper or a soft cloth.

Sparkling Window Cleaner

1	Tablespoon vinegar	1	Teaspoon cornstarch
1	Tablespoon ammonia	2	Drops liquid detergent

Add 1 cup water and store in a pump spray bottle. Shake before spraying onto windows, then wipe off with wadded up newspaper.

Window Cloth

Make your own instant window cleaner cloth! Combine 1/2 teaspoon liquid soap, 1/4 cup vinegar, and 2 cups water. Soak a sponge or small cloth in this mixture, then wring it out. Store the window cloth in a glass jar with a tight fitting lid until needed. Then simply wipe spots and smears from dirty windows. They will clean up without streaks - no mess, no fuss.

Mirrors

To clean mirrors, spray a vinegar and water solution onto a cloth, then wipe the mirror with the cloth. Never spray ANY liquid onto a mirror. Dampness can get to the silvering on the mirror's back and cause it to flake, peel away or discolor.

Mop Magic

For stay-shiny-longer floors, make this special glossy surface cleaning solution. To a bucket of warm water, add 1/2 cup fabric softener and 1/4 cup vinegar. Mop as usual and watch the magic shine appear. This works best for lightly soiled floors.

Waxed Surfaces

Clean waxed surfaces with vinegar, instead of ammonia-based products, because ammonia dissolves wax. Also, use cool water to keep the wax hard. Hot water softens wax and makes it easier for tiny particles of dirt to become embedded in it, rather than being washed off.

Waxing Floors

Make your floor wax go on smoother, last longer and shine brighter by rinsing the floor with a strong solution of water and white vinegar before applying wax. A cup of vinegar to a half bucket of warm water is about right.

Quick Pick-Up For No-Wax Floors

Mix white vinegar and water, half and half, in a pump spray bottle. Mist the traffic areas of no-wax flooring and immediately buff dry with an old towel. This quick pickup will have the floor looking shiny clean in about two minutes!

Really Dirty Vinyl Floors

Pre-treating really dirty vinyl floors can make the job of cleaning them easier. Spray full strength vinegar on spots, globs and sticky areas. Let set for 5 minutes, then mop as usual.

Scented Air Freshener

Fill a pump spray bottle with well-strained herbal vinegar and use a few puffs to both cleanse the air and to add refreshing, natural scents. Often these scented air fresheners do not cause the allergic sniffles and sneezes some people experience when using commercial fresheners.

Urine Stained Mattresses

Spray stains with white vinegar and blot dry. The process may need to be repeated several times, but it should eventually lift most stains and unpleasant odors.

Freshen Bedding

Musty, stale smelling blankets and bedspreads can be freshened, often without actually having to clean or wash them. Simply put the bedding in a clothes dryer with a cloth wrung out of full strength apple cider vinegar. With the dryer set to 'air,' let it fluff for 5 minutes. Most odors and dust will disappear and the apple cider vinegar will leave a clean, outdoorsy smell behind. Dusty drapes can be refreshed in the same manner.

Books

After awhile, even the nicest books can develop a musty smell. Keep them spotlessly clean by running a vacuum cleaner over them frequently. If individual volumes need to be hand dusted, try wiping the covers with a soft cloth which has been very lightly sprayed with a weak vinegar and water solution. (You only want enough vinegar to kill the musty smell and to deter mold and fungus growth.)

Bookshelves

Use a strong solution of vinegar and sudsy water to wipe off book-shelves, then rinse in clear water and dry. Make shelf cleaning less exhausting by only removing 4 or 5 books from a shelf. Wash and dry the exposed part of the shelf, then slide the next 4 or 5 books over this clean spot and wash the part now exposed.

Repeat the process to the end of the shelf. When the entire shelf has been washed and dried, slide the books back to their original positions and replace the few books that were removed at the beginning. This way, lifting of heavy books is minimized for the one doing the cleaning, shelf order is maintained, and the books do not suffer unnecessary handling.

Window Shades and Blinds

Keep shades and blinds clean and free of smudges by wiping them down regularly with a cloth dampened in a mild vinegar and sudsy water solution.

Another Furniture Polish

When 1/4 cup linseed oil, 1/8 cup vinegar, and 1/8 cup whiskey are mixed together, they make a nice furniture polish. Dirt seems to disappear as the alcohol evaporates.

Metal Cleaner

Make a good metal cleaner by combining 2 tablespoons cream of tartar and enough vinegar to make a paste. Rub it on and let it dry. Wash it off with plain warm water and dry with an old towel. Metal will gleam.

Doorknobs

Some of the dirtiest places in the home (and most forgotten hiding places for germs) are the doorknobs. Most will benefit from an occasional cleaning with a cloth dampened in vinegar. It will kill germs and wipe away dirt. Glass doorknobs will sparkle like new!

Sanitize The Telephone

Germs that cause colds and flu live on surfaces that are handled by many different members of the household. Prevent germs from spreading from one person to another by wiping the telephone receiver down with full strength vinegar to kill any bacteria that may be breeding on it.

VINEGAR IN THE LAUNDRY

About 3000 B.C. cotton fabric was first made in the Indus valley, about 400 B.C. laundry was still washed in a stream. In 1625 soap was made at home by boiling grease, fat and wood ashes; by 1837 Procter & Gamble™ began selling mass produced soap. A popular homemaker's advice book of 1849 admonished the housekeeper to "Remove soil spots with equal parts vinegar, turpentine and linseed oil." And, "Boil soiled laundry for 20 minutes in water with soap, lye, sal soda, and turpentine."

In 1907 Thor, the first completely self-contained electric washing machine was introduced by Hurley Machine Company of Chicago and soon after, in 1907 Persil, the first dishwashing detergent, came on the market. (Unfortunately, it was not suitable for heavy duty laundry use.)

In 1922 Maytag's® Gyrofoam washing machine was a market star and in 1934 the first Washeteria (laundromat) opened in Fort Worth, Texas with four washing machines. Finally, in 1946 Procter & Gamble™ introduced Tide®, the first detergent strong enough for washing clothes was introduced.

Wash day has changed! Today's fabrics are often delicate, and require gentle cleaning. As the washing of clothes left river banks and soap gave way to detergent, standards of cleanliness changed, too. Now, laundry is expected to be more than clean. Whites must gleam and colors need to sparkle.

Surface tension is what lets a water spider walk on water.

Fabrics that come through the laundry room may be synthetic or natural, delicate or sturdy, drab or iridescent, easily faded or colorfast. This parade of materials, textures, fibers and dyes presents difficult cleaning choices — does one use soap or detergent? Bleach, an alkaline washing booster, an enzymatic prewash or vinegar? Understanding how laundry cleaning substances do their jobs can help you decide when to use soap, when to use detergent and when to use vinegar as a cleaning agent.

SOAP OR DETERGENT?

Soaps clean by encouraging tiny bits of dirt to become solid curds that can be rinsed out by water. Soap leaves a light, oily film behind that attracts more dirt to fabrics.

Detergents include an ingredient to make water 'wet' better by breaking its surface tension. This lets it do a better job of dissolving dirt out of fabrics. Detergents also contain emulsifiers, which help to keep the bits of dirt suspended in water. Rinsing in lots of water helps get rid of this dirt, too. Most soaps and detergents are alkaline. Vinegar's acid nature makes it a good neutralizing rinse for laundry washed in either soap or detergent.

Use vinegar with care. Vinegar has been considered, throughout history, to be an indispensable part of cleaning laundry. This is because it is often the best product for rinsing natural fibers. It is not always as compatible with synthetic fibers. There are some fabrics for which vinegar is not appropriate. For example, in some situations vinegar acts as a mild bleaching agent. So, before applying it to dark or bright colors, test it on small, hidden areas. And, because vinegar is an acid, it can intensify the actions of other acids, making it a poor choice for treating some man-made fibers.

143

Generally, silk and wool can take a dash of full strength white vinegar. For fine cottons and linens, use vinegar that has been diluted with an equal amount of water, as it can weaken these fibers. Acetate and triacetate are cellulose based and should not be exposed to vinegar at all. Triacetate is the material that is often used for lightweight, finely pleated skirts. Ramie, a plant fiber based material, is not helped by vinegar either. (When cellulose products decompose they turn into something much like vinegar!).

USE VINEGAR TO NEUTRALIZE ALKALINES

Vinegar is particularly good at neutralizing alkaline stains. So, use vinegar to neutralize the effects of caustic products, such as dishwasher detergents and solutions containing lye, such as oven cleaners. This means vinegar can be very helpful as a neutralizing rinse for hands exposed to caustic alkaline cleaners. And, use vinegar on stains made by: syrup, food dye, apples, blueberries, jelly, hair colorings, pears, grapefruit, honey, spaghetti, cherries, blackberries, oranges, perfume, grapes, raspberries

Vinegar is useful for removing many of the discolorations caused by medicines, inks and fabric dyes. It is also good for lifting traces of beer, wine, grass, soft drinks, coffee, tea and tobacco. Ammonia is very alkaline and can alter the color of some dyes; stop this change in color by neutralizing the action of ammonia with vinegar. When fabric begins to bleed color because it has been exposed to ammonia, rinse it in cool water. Follow with a strong vinegar and water solution, then finish with a clear water rinse.

One of the few stains vinegar should not be used on, is one caused by blood. Vinegar can set it and make it nearly impossible to get out. (See Spit & Polish, near the end of this chapter, for vinegar's contribution to removing blood stains.) Do not use vinegar on stains made by: blood, vomit, eggs, butter, milk or grease.

Pre-Treating Solution
4 Tablespoons vinegar
2 Tablespoons baking soda
3 Tablespoons ammonia
Cool water
1 Tablespoon liquid detergent
Many laundry stains may be removed by pre-treating clothes with a few spritzes of this stain remover. To make, put the vinegar, ammonia, and liquid detergent in a quart-size pump spray bottle. Mix together, then add the baking soda. When it stops foaming, fill the bottle with cool water and use immediately. (If the mixture is stored in this container, the pump spray may be damaged.)

Laundry Booster

1/4 cup vinegar added to a load of laundry, along with the usual soap, will brighten colors and make whites sparkle. This will also act as a fabric softener, and inhibit mold and fungus growth. It helps to kill athlete's foot germs on socks, too.

New Clothes

Vinegar is a good addition to the laundry tub when new clothes are being washed for the first time. It will help to eliminate possibly irritating manufacturing chemicals and their odors.

General Perspiration Stains

White vinegar is the traditional remedy for removing perspiration stains from clothes. Sturdy fabrics can be treated with a full strength application of vinegar, rubbed in as they are put in the washing machine. Delicate fabrics should be soaked in vinegar diluted half and half with water.

Stubborn Perspiration Stains

White fabric that has been stained by perspiration can sometimes be cleaned with white vinegar, salt and lots of sunlight. Begin by wringing the entire garment out in cool water. Then soak the stains with full strength white vinegar. Spread the clothing out in direct sunlight and sprinkle the stain with salt. When the garment is completely dry, repeat the process. Most perspiration stains will eventually come out this way.

Use white vinegar to remove stains.

Perspiration and Silks

Delicate silk garments are notorious for attracting perspiration stains.

White vinegar is the safest, surest way to pre-treat this kind of discoloration. Many silks can tolerate a brief splash of full strength white vinegar to underarm areas without harm. (As always, test on an inconspicuous area before using any stain treatment!) To begin, wet the entire garment, then apply white vinegar to discolored underarm stains. Let set for 3 minutes (longer on sturdy, colorfast fabrics and some whites). Wash as usual, being sure to add a dash of white vinegar to the final rinse water.

Keep Silks Shiny

To help silk garments keep their soft shine, always include a dash of white vinegar in their last rinse water. It helps them retain their glossy sheen.

Easy White Vinegar Rinse

An easy way to add vinegar to the last rinse water is to soak several white washcloths in full strength white vinegar and store them in a closed container. Then, just toss one of these prepared cloths into the rinse water when the washer tub has filled. It saves measuring and eliminates the possibility of splashing vinegar directly onto delicate fabrics.

Static Cling Solution

Make your own dryer sheets by preparing several small cloths wrung out of full strength white vinegar (as above). Then, simply toss a damp cloth into the dryer with each load of laundry. (This is also a good way to freshen and soften clothes if you forget to add vinegar to the last rinse cycle!)

Static Cling

Fight static cling in the dryer with nylon fabric and vinegar. Simply spray a 2 foot square of nylon net with a half and half solution of white vinegar and water and add it to a dryer load of clothes. The nylon net square will not only help reduce static cling, it will collect lint.

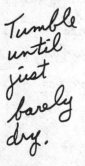

Tumble until just barely dry.

Warmer Blankets

The fluff on the blanket is what makes it keep you warm. The softer and fluffier the blanket, the better job it will do of keeping you warm. Spray lots of white vinegar on blankets before drying them. It will help to make them soft and fluffy. (Or, add the vinegar to the rinse water.)

Ink Stains

Ink stains can often be lifted by soaking them in white vinegar. Put full strength vinegar on ink stains, allow to set for 15 seconds then blot. Repeat several times for dark stains, then wash as usual. Or, soak clothes in milk for an hour. Then cover the stain with a paste of vinegar and cornstarch. When the paste dries, wash the garment as usual.

Coffee & Tea Stains

Blot splatters until as much as possible of the liquid is removed. Immediately rinse in cool water. Follow with a rinse of white vinegar then wash in lukewarm, soapy water.

Stubborn Coffee and Tea Stains

Coffee or tea stains that are very dark, or those that have been allowed to set, require extra treatment. Dampen the stain with white vinegar and sprinkle it with salt. Then, expose the stain to bright sunlight for at least an hour. Follow this by washing the material as usual. Repeat the process as necessary.

Red Wine Stains

Blot spills thoroughly, then immediately rinse the area with white wine. Blot again, until nearly dry, then rinse several times with white vinegar. Wash with mild suds and check to see if any discoloration remains. If further treatment is needed, soak in vinegar, then wash again in soapy water before drying.

Rust Stains

Rust marks on cloth can usually be lifted with white vinegar and salt. Simply wet the rust stain with vinegar and then cover it with salt. Let it dry, preferably in the sun. Rinse the salt out and reapply until the stain is gone.

Basic Fabric Softener

Add 1/3 cup white vinegar to the final rinse water for softer, scent-free laundry. This inexpensive laundry treatment is safe for the gentlest fabrics and is great for those who are allergic to harsh chemicals and strong scents.

Amazing Fabric Softener

Combine 1/3 cup white vinegar and 1/3 cup baking soda and add the mixture to the final rinse water for even softer laundry. This combination is scent-free and irritation-free, good for the most delicate skin and fabrics. Softener Hint: Keep vinegar-based fabric softeners in a pump spray bottle, such as liquid hand soap comes in. Then just add a few squirts to laundry water. No muss, no fuss!

Scented Fabric Softener

To add a very faint hint of clean, outdoorsy smell to laundry, use apple cider in any of the previous fabric softeners. For stronger scents, use herbal vinegars, such as lavender or rose.

Lint Trap

Hard water can cause a buildup of minerals on the lint trap of the washing machine. Soak it in full strength vinegar for a couple of hours, then use a brush to remove the deposits.

Pantyhose Revitalizer

Soak stretched out, shapeless pantyhose in 1 quart of warm water, with 1/4 cup white vinegar added to it. Let them set for 5 minutes, then squeeze gently and blot with a bath towel. (Never wring or stretch wet hose.) Allow the pantyhose to dry, spread out flat on a towel.

Brightener For Synthetics

When polyester or nylon fabrics have become dull and drab looking, boiling them in 2 quarts of water, with 3/4 cup white vinegar added to it, can sometimes revitalize them.

Protecting Wool

Harsh alkaline laundry products can easily damage good wools, as well as silks. For many hundreds of years white vinegar has been the cleaning fluid of choice for these fabrics. It helps to keep them soft, while lifting odors and stains. This will also protect colors by preventing a buildup of soap or detergent residues.

Renewing Wool Apparel

Add new life to wool garments whose cuffs, bottoms or necklines have become stretched out and have lost their ability to snap back into their original shape. Combine vinegar and heat to recondition these wool clothes. Add 2 tablespoons of white vinegar to a small bucket of very hot water. Carefully dip only the stretched out edge of the garment into the hot water. Immediately blot with a towel and blow dry with a hair dryer set on its highest setting.

Mohair is another name for angora.

Alpaca

Alpaca is a wool-like fiber from llamas. This material will hold its shape and remain soft and springy for many years if rinsed in water with a tablespoon of white vinegar in it.

Camel Hair Wool

This is an exceptional soft and silky kind of wool. Wash it in gentle suds, rinse in a dilute water and vinegar solution, and dry on a flat surface.

Angora

Angora has a texture much like that of fine lamb's wool. It can be made from the fur of angora rabbits or goats. It responds well to a gentle washing, followed by a rinse in cool water with a couple of tablespoons of white vinegar mixed in.

Cashmere

This wool is named after the goat whose undercoat provides the hair it is made of. Originally found in Kashmir, Tibet, these goats are now raised in many other areas. Treat cashmere as any good wool.

Fresh Smelling Linens

Remove stale odors from linens by spraying them, lightly, with vinegar water, then fluffing them in the dryer for 5 or 10 minutes. (To a 1 quart pump spray bottle of water, add 1 or 2 tablespoons of white vinegar.) Or, put the dry linens in the dryer with a vinegar and water dampened bath towel.

Long Lasting Creases For Pants

No-iron cotton pants will hold a sharp crease if treated with wax and vinegar. Begin by turning the pants inside out. Then run the bottom of a wax candle down the crease line (on the wrong side of the fabric). Next, turn the pants right side out and cover the crease line with a cloth wrung out of half water, half white vinegar. Press with a very hot iron until dry. The crease will be sharp, and it will stay that way for a long time!

Wrinkle Remover

Remove wrinkles from stored clothes by hanging them in the bathroom. Put 1 cup vinegar in the bath tub and turn the hot water in the shower on. When the tub is 1/2 full, turn off the water and allow the clothes to hang in the steamy room for 20 minutes. Most wrinkles will be removed and any stale odors will be gone, too.

Reviving Straw Hats

Stained and misshapen straw hats can be revived with a vinegar and salt treatment. Stir 1/2 cup salt into a large bucket or laundry tub of warm water. When the salt is dissolved, submerge the hat in the water. When the straw is soft, gently wipe away any stains, using a little liquid soap if necessary. Remove the hat from the water and allow to drain for a few minutes. Gently push it into the desired shape, then spray the hat with a fine mist of vinegar water. (Add 1 teaspoon white vinegar to 1 cup water.) Allow to dry, away from the sun.

Crystal Clear Leather Cleaner

1/4 Cup white vinegar   1 Cup water
1/4 Cup rubbing alcohol

Gently wipe leather with a cloth dampened in this clear leather cleaner and dry at once with another cloth. This cleaner also works well on leather look-alike fabrics.

Curtains and Sheer Panels

Revitalize delicate fabric window coverings by using this vinegar based treatment in the final rinse. To a quart of hot water, add 1 tablespoon white vinegar and 2 envelopes of plain (unsweetened, unflavored) gelatin. Add this mixture to the final rinse water and dry as usual. Limp fabrics will be instantly revitalized!

Removing Gum

Break up sticky gum residue by soaking it in white vinegar. Begin by scraping away as much of the gum as possible. Then pat white vinegar onto what remains and let set for 20 minutes. Blot the vinegar away, taking as much of the gum with it as possible. Repeat until all the gum is gone.

Spit & Polish

For one of the best ways vinegar can help remove stains, it does not even need to touch the stain! Stains made by dairy products such as milk, eggs and cream are best dissolved by special digestive enzymes — the kind of enzymes found in human spit. To lift these stains, place a few tablespoons of apple cider vinegar in a small bowl and breathe the vapor that rises from it. This will encourage digestive juices to flow, ensuring plenty of spit for soaking away stains. Small drops of blood or wine that have left spots on cloth can often be removed this way, and some kinds of grease, too.

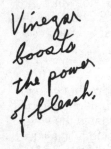
Vinegar boosts the power of bleach.

Pretty Red Dye

1/2	Cup vinegar	1	Pound beets
1	Quart water		

Wash a pound of fresh beets and place them, with their skins on, in a sauce pan and cover with cool water. Simmer until the beets are tender, then remove skins. Chop the beets and return them to the same water in which they were cooked. Let them set for 2 hours, then strain off the liquid and add the vinegar. Use this liquid to turn cloth a warm, rose color.

Please remember! Always test fabrics and surfaces before using even a gentle cleaner like vinegar. No one cleaner is perfect for every laundry chore. Vinegar's antibacterial, antiseptic, and mild bleaching actions, as well as its acid nature may not be perfectly safe for every fabric. As with all cleaning substances, your own test on fabrics is the only sure test of safety.

MISCELLANEOUS

Vinegar also has terrific versatility as a cleaner and neutralizer of caustic substances. On the pages that follow, you will see its usefulness on shoes, furniture, floors, luggage and much more!

Taking The White Out

White correction fluid is wonderful stuff, until it shows up where it is not needed! Usually, a quick dab of white vinegar will melt it away. (For stubborn spots, reapply or soak for a few minutes.)

Super-Glued Fingers

When an errant drop of one of those new fast drying contact glues gets on skin, fingers can end up cemented together. For a skin saving remedy, soak them in full strength vinegar.

Colored Paper Stains
Vivid shades of construction paper can brighten up office projects, but a little dampness can cause bright colors to transfer onto clothing. Lift these stains by dampening with a solution of half white vinegar, half water, then blot dry. Repeat until all trace of color is gone.

Renew Suede Shoes
Put 2 cups water and 1/4 cup white vinegar in a pan and heat to the boiling point. Set heat to simmer and, while holding each shoe in the steam, gently brush up the nap. Set the shoes aside until completely dry before wearing.

Stay-Tied Trick For Leather Shoelaces
Leather shoestrings are notorious for their inability to hold a knot. The next time you want leather shoelaces to stay tied, put 3 drops of apple cider vinegar on the knot and give it an extra tug. The laces will stay tied until you untie them.

End Squeaky Floors
Quiet noisy wooden floors by forcing a mixture of vinegar and liquid soap into the cracks between boards. To each cup of liquid soap, add 2 tablespoons vinegar and mix well.

Old-Fashioned Wallpaper Paste
1/2 Cup cornstarch   6 Cups boiling water
3/4 Cup cold water   1/4 Cup white vinegar
Mix cornstarch and cold water and stir, all at once, into boiling water. When the mixture boils again remove from heat, pour through a strainer and stir in the vinegar. (This also makes a great laundry starch!)

Tape Remover
A compress of vinegar will loosen the sticky glue on adhesive bandages, making removal less painful. Vinegar also softens the adhesives on masking, duct, strapping and other tapes.

Glue Removal
Most glues can be softened by soaking them in full strength vinegar.

Add a drop of liquid detergent to help vinegar penetrate faster.

Better Humidifying
Add a couple of tablespoons of white vinegar to the water in a humidifier to eliminate odors in the home. Vinegar will also discourage

the growth of germs in the humidifier's water reservoir.

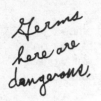
Germs here are dangerous!

Cleaning the Humidifier
At least once a week, soak the water reservoir for 10 minutes in a solution of 1 part white vinegar to 10 parts water. The vinegar will help to dissolve minerals salts, allowing them to be washed out so there is no buildup on the inside of the humidifier.

Instant Humidifying
Keep a spray filled with water that has a splash of white vinegar added to it. Whenever the air in a room is too dry, several pumps of the sprayer will provide an instant improvement in the humidity level.

Cleaning the Dehumidifier
Clean the water collecting tray with a brush dipped in full strength vinegar. If it is cleaned regularly, minerals will not build up in the tray and clog the outlet. Add a splash of white vinegar to the water collecting tray to discourage the growth of germs and to keep the water from smelling stale and mildewy.

The fish will thank you.

Aquariums
A mild vinegar and water solution is the ideal substance for cleaning the outside of glass aquariums. Spray a soft cloth with a weak vinegar and water mixture (1 cup water, 1 teaspoon vinegar) and wipe surfaces until completely dry. Very dirty aquarium glass can be scrubbed with a cloth wrung out of full strength vinegar. Rub dry with a soft cloth. Never spray aquarium glass, because fine droplets of mist can settle into the water and disrupt its the delicate ph balance.

Wallpaper Stripper
To each cup of vinegar, add 1 tablespoon liquid detergent. Spray or wipe this solution onto walls and allow it to set a few minutes. Most papers will scrape off easily.

Wood Scratches
Repair scratches in wood furniture with vinegar and a fresh walnut! Wipe the scratched area with a cloth dampened in full strength vinegar. Crack open a walnut and immediately rub the scratch with a piece of the kernel. Wood scratches can also be repaired with vinegar and iodine. Mix equal parts of each in a small dish and apply with an artist's paintbrush. Add extra iodine for a deeper color, more vinegar for a lighter color.

Molded Plastic Luggage

Hard-sided suitcases can be cleaned with a solution made of half gentle liquid detergent and half white vinegar. Follow with a clear water rinse before buffing dry. Remember, handles need cleaning, too.

Saddle Soap

A good saddle soap can be made from 1/8 cup liquid soap, 1/8 cup linseed oil, 1/4 cup beeswax, and 1/4 cup vinegar. Warm the beeswax, slowly, in the vinegar. Then add the soap and oil. Keep the mixture warm until it will all mix together smoothly. Then cool until it is solid. To use, rub it onto good leather, then buff to a high shine.

Leather Polish

Polish leather with a mixture of 2/3 cup linseed oil, 1/3 cup vinegar, and 1/3 cup water. Beat it all together and apply with a soft cloth. Then buff with a clean rag.

Glue-Be-Gone

Most any old wood glue can be softened for easy removal. Simply wet the glued area down with vinegar, and keep it wet overnight. Even some of the newfangled super-duper hold-it-all glues can be scraped away if they are soaked overnight in vinegar.

Play-Clay

1	Cup flour	1 Teaspoon vinegar
1/2	Cup salt	1 Tablespoon oil
1	Cup water	

Just for fun.

Combine all ingredients in a saucepan and heat. Stir continually, until it forms a ball. Remove from heat, allow to cool, then knead until smooth. A few drops of food coloring may be worked into it while kneading. Store between uses in a tightly sealed container in the refrigerator.

CAUTION

ALWAYS test a small, inconspicuous area of fabrics, wall coverings, flooring, etc. before using any cleaning product — including vinegar. No product, even one as safe and gentle as vinegar, is safe for every person or every situation. While vinegar has been safely used for thousands of years, it is possible for certain individuals to be sensitive to it. If there is any possibility that you may be sensitive or allergic to vinegar, consult a medical professional before exposing your skin to it.

When cleaning copper, always dispose of all cleaning cloths or paper towels as soon as the job is finished — that green tarnish on copper is poisonous!

Vinegar Goes Outside

Vinegar is exceptionally useful in the garden, yard and garage. For cleaning and polishing, or for deterring insects, it is difficult to find a better, more environmentally safe substance. Vinegar is a gentle, inexpensive cleaner, yet it is surprisingly effective. It is safe for children and pets, yet it attacks germs and harmful bacteria. Whether shining and polishing the car or washing the dog, there is usually a good reason to keep the vinegar bottle handy!

OUTSIDE THE HOUSE

Home Ant Repellant

Sprinkle apple cider vinegar on windowsills and around doors and other openings to prevent ants from entering the home.

Peel-No-More Painting

Concrete walls and floors will take a coat of paint without troublesome peeling if the surface is first painted with vinegar. Brush on the vinegar, let the concrete dry, then paint as usual. This works on metal, too!

Paint Brush Renewal

Old, stiff paint brushes can be restored to their former softness by removing dried-in paint. Simply put paint stiffened brushes in a small saucepan and cover them with full strength vinegar. Bring to a boil and simmer for 15 minutes. When cool enough to touch, work the softened paint out of the bristles under hot running water. Repeat as necessary. (Wood handled brushes are better candidates then plastic handled ones which may distort when heated.) Dry paint brushes by shaking them or spinning them between your palms. Do not stand brushes on their bristles, as that will ruin their shape.

Painted Windows

Make removing paint from window glass easier by mixing a good, thick liquid detergent half and half with white vinegar. Spread this over the paint and allow to almost dry before removing the paint with a scraper. The thick detergent helps keep the vinegar from running off and together they soften the paint.

Wet-Dry Vac

Half fill a pail with warm water and a cup of vinegar. Suck this solution up into the shop vac to clean and deodorize it. Let the warm liquid set for 3 minutes, then dump the water out and wipe the inside of the vac clean. Allow to air dry before putting it back together. Keeping the unit clean will extend the life of filters and prevent foul odors.

Barbecue Grills

Place soiled racks from barbecue grills in a large black plastic bag. Use 2 cups of vinegar to wet them down, then tie a loose knot in the bag to seal in the moisture. Lay the plastic bag in the sun for 3 to 4 hours, then add 2 tablespoons dishwasher detergent and 2 quarts hot water to it. Re-tie the bag and allow it to soak in the sun for another 2 hours. Burnt food and stains will now wipe off easily.

Cement Garage Floors

Sweeping cement can produce a fine dust that is very corrosive. Reduce dust with newspapers and vinegar water. To a gallon of water, add 1 cup vinegar. Sprinkle this liberally over a pile of shredded newspapers. Toss the shredded newspapers over the floor, then sweep as usual. Dust will cling to the damp newspaper and the vinegar will help neutralize odors.

Vinegar foams when added to dry soil with a high ph.

Green Sweep For Cement Floors

Cut down on dust when sweeping cement floors by spreading grass clippings over the floor (the fresher the better). Dampen the clippings by sprinkling with water that has had a little apple cider vinegar added to it. The sweeping will not generate dust, and when the job is done, the area will smell fresh and clean!

Broom Revitalizer

Old plastic brooms (and cornstalk ones, too) can be reshaped and deodorized by soaking them in a bucket of very hot water to which a cup of apple cider vinegar has been added. Let the bristles soak for at least 10 minutes, then shake the broom to remove most of the water. Wrap two or three large rubber bands around the bristles and set the broom in the sun for several hours. When the rubber bands are removed the broom will retain its new, neat shape. And best of all, it will smell fresh and clean!

'New' Stubby Broom

When a broom is finally ready to be discarded, try cutting about half the length of the bristles off. Angle the cut so that the bristles on the short side are about 1 inch in length and the ones on the long side about are about 5 inches in length. Soak the broom as above, shake it out and set in the sun until dry. This 'new' stubby broom will do a great job in corners and other places that are hard to reach with a regular broom. And, the long handle will save the bending and crawling that using a regular whisk broom requires.

Film-Free Window Washing

Outside windows that have their frames painted with latex paint, and windows in homes where the siding is painted with latex paint, often pick up a cloudy film. This is because of the natural sloughing-off process of this kind of paint. Soaps and detergents do not dissolve this fine coating of latex. Rinsing windows in water with lots of white vinegar in it neutralizes the film and helps to keep the glass clear and clean.

Old Windows

When window glass seems dull and 'old' looking, it is usually because soap scum and hard water minerals have been allowed to build up on it. Vinegar is very good at cutting through the haze and restoring the shine to such window glass.

Streaky Windows

Streaks on windows are usually caused by the sun heating the glass and making the cleaning solution dry too fast. Wash windows on a cloudy day to minimize sun streaking. Or, wash windows on the shady side of the house, then wait for the sun to move. Using a squeegee to remove the cleaning solution will also minimize streaking.

Sharpen Knives

Need to sharpen a knife in a hurry? Spray vinegar onto

the bottom of a clay flowerpot. Then use the edge of the pot as a whetstone.

Sponges
Cleanup sponges can be renewed and made to feel new by washing them in vinegar water, then soaking them overnight in 1 quart of water with 1/4 cup vinegar added to it.

Metal
Use vinegar to clean away mineral buildup on metal. Just add 1/4 cup to a quart of water for cleaning metal screen and storm doors and aluminum furniture. Add extra vinegar if your water has a particularly high mineral content.

IN THE GARDEN

Gardener's Friend
Keep ants away from plants by making a circle around them with vinegar. Just dribble a generous stream around each plant; it will act as a barrier to wandering ants.

Flowerpots
After a very short time the outsides of clay flowerpots can develop a buildup of mineral salts. This whitish film not only looks ugly, it interferes with the way the pot should breathe and absorb water. Remove mineral salts by rubbing with a scrub brush dipped in full strength vinegar. Finish with a clear water rinse.

Soil Ph Balancer
Many plants need an acid soil environment to thrive. To acidify alkaline ground, pour 1 cup vinegar into a bucket of water and dribble it in a circle around acid loving plants such as azaleas, blueberries, marigolds and radishes.

FOR THE CAR

Odor-Eater For Car Ashtrays
Wipe ashtrays out with a wadded up newspaper or paper towel moistened with full strength vinegar. Allow to air dry. The vinegar will neutralize ashtray odor, and as it dries it will remove stale smells from the entire car.

No-Freeze, No-Streak Windshield Washer Liquid

1/2 Cup white vinegar
2 Cups rubbing alcohol
2 Teaspoons liquid detergent
6 Cups water

Stir the detergent in the water and when it is well mixed, add the vinegar and alcohol. This liquid will also help remove ice and snow from a cold car's windshield. Simply spray a good coating on before trying to clear the windshield of ice. It will make the job much easier.

Chrome Cleaner

Remove small spots of rust from car chrome by rubbing them out with a piece of aluminum foil dipped in vinegar. Rinse, and then finish up with a coat of wax to discourage new spots from forming.

Decal Remover

Soak bumper decals in full strength white vinegar and they will come off easily. Just wrap a cloth around the bumper, wet it thoroughly with vinegar, then allow it to set for 45 minutes. The glue holding the decal to the bumper should begin to break down, making removal much easier!

Boat Cleaning

Aluminum boats, in particular, are very sensitive to alkalines in water. These salts can etch aluminum and cause it to discolor. Vinegar neutralizes alkalines, so it can be used to scrub off discoloration. Use full strength white vinegar to scrub stains, but always follow with a clear water rinse, then immediately wipe dry.

ESPECIALLY FOR CAMPERS

No-Scrub Laundry

Do laundry while on the road by placing soiled clothes in a watertight container with a tiny bit of detergent and some white vinegar. After a few hours on the road the laundry will be ready to rinse and hang out to dry!

Vacation Skin

Always tuck a bottle of vinegar into the camping pack. It is great for soothing skin that has been subjected to sun and wind. It is also good for softening hard water.

Fiberglass Campers

Because it is light in weight, many camping trailers use fiberglass for both exterior and interior surfaces. This material tends to pickup hard water stains and soap scum film. White vinegar helps dissolve this whitish discoloration. Use it on fiberglass sinks, wall panels, tubs and showers.

Plastic Picnic Coolers

Spray a strong vinegar and detergent solution over the inside of the cooler. Close it up to soak while you wash the outside of the cooler with vinegar and water. By the time you get to the inside, odors and food remains will wipe right off.

PETS

Animals need vinegar, too. Vinegar can be as important to animals as it is to people. It freshens drinking water, shines coats, discourages parasites and fights infections. Some of the remedies for pets, pests and nuisances that appear in this chapter have been validated by the latest scientific findings. Others are based on long-standing tradition and folk wisdom. For your safety, and that of your pets and farm animals, ALWAYS CHECK WITH YOUR VETERINARIAN BEFORE TREATING ANIMALS WITH HOME REMEDIES!

Itch Control For Dogs

Help to control itching by following the dog's bath with a vinegar and water rinse. Add 1/3 cup apple cider vinegar to 2 quarts water and pour over a well shampooed and rinsed dog. Do not rinse out. Dry as usual and the coat should be soft and shiny, and there should be much less itching and scratching.

Odor Control

Control odor from any furry pet by spraying its coat daily with mild vinegar water. One tablespoon to a cup of water is about right for eliminating odors.

Behavior Control

Train cats and dogs to respect furniture with a squirt gun filled with water that has a teaspoon of vinegar added to it. Whenever the pet approaches a forbidden area tell them NO and reinforce it with a quick liquid reminder. Soon, simply picking up the squirt gun will ensure good behavior.

Carpet Spots

Use a solution made of 1 cup white vinegar to a gallon of lukewarm water to neutralize urine stains in carpet. Sprinkle it on, then immediately blot it up. Repeat as needed.

Pet Hair

Turn an old tube sock inside out and slip in onto your hand. Spray it, lightly, with white vinegar and use it to wipe down your pet; loose hair will stick to the damp sock. Great for cats, dogs, hamsters, rabbits and other furry creatures. It also deodorizes their fur. A vinegar dampened sock is also good for removing pet hairs from furniture, carpets and clothing.

Vinegar Is For Birds, Too!

Keep birdbaths clean by rinsing them out regularly. A few drops of vinegar added to birdbath water will help control the growth of fungus and bacteria.

Through The Year With Vinegar

*B*its of vinegar history, cleaning tips, folklore and the very best old-time home remedies – that is what you will find as you go through the year with vinegar!

January

1

Chinese doctors have found vaporized vinegar useful against flu germs. This may help to explain the usefulness of old-time remedies that suggested sniffing vinegar to avoid diseases such as the plague.

2

Italy of olden times was known for an all-purpose sauce that was used at most meals. The salted entrails of fish were aged in vinegar to make a distinctive, strong smelling, condiment.

3

Egyptians considered vinegar to be an appetite stimulant, so they value it as part of huge banquets.

4

It has long been believed that patting apple cider vinegar onto the feet will decrease foot odors. This seems to work because apple cider vinegar gets its color from enzymatic browning of apples, which energizes natural tannins in the fruit. These compounds have astringent qualities that can help control perspiration odor on feet.

5

During the U.S. Civil War vinegar was sipped by soldiers, on both sides of the conflict, to guard against scurvy.

6

Put fresh honeysuckle blossoms in hot vinegar and age the mixture for at least two or three weeks. The result will be a fragrant elixir used by our grandmothers to clear away freckles. It will also ease the sting of a mild sun or windburn.

7

The Roman Emperor, Tiberius, is reputed to have liked the taste of cucumbers with a vinegar and honey dressing. He is said to have eaten this dish with lots of pepper sprinkled over it.

8

Many years ago, apple cider vinegar was considered a beneficial liquid for cleaning the teeth and strengthening the gums. We now know too frequent use could damage tooth enamel. So, always rinse after using vinegar in the mouth. If you drink an apple cider vinegar tonic every day, use a straw to protect your teeth from vinegar's acid.

9

For many years apple cider vinegar and cornstarch have been used as a paste to ease the pain of shingles.

10

In Traditional Chinese Medicine those with hepatitis are given sugar-sweetened vinegar that has had pork bones boiled in it to relieve the accompanying jaundice.

11

When vinegar is made in the old-fashioned, 'natural' way, a thick, sticky mass called "mother" forms on top of the liquid and aids in the fermentation process. The technical term for mother is Zoogloea mycoderma.

12

Bits of the sticky mass that forms during vinegar making (called mother) are often transferred from one batch of vinegar to another, as a starter for the new batch. Old world vinegar makers guard this valuable starter because it helps retain the uniqueness of each producer's vinegar.

13

Before apples are used to make apple cider vinegar, it is very important that they are thoroughly washed to remove any chemicals that may have been sprayed on the ripening apples. One of these chemicals is Alar, a chemical which is used to control the time frame in which apples grow and ripen. It is a brand name for daminozide, a chemical that, during processing, changes into UDMH (a substance chemically related to rocket fuel). Scientists feel it is most probably a carcinogen to which children are especially vulnerable.

14

Pasteurized vinegar, if the bottle is not opened, will retain its goodness for years. Once the bottle has been opened it will begin to lose a little of its zip in about 3 months, even if kept tightly capped.

15

An old Italian dish was made by salting purslane, then covering it with vinegar. This was a good way to preserve a green vegetable for winter eating.

16

Vinegar with lemon slices in it is a good skin astringent that reduces the redness and prickling of sunburn.

17

Although some other countries produce a vinegar they refer to as balsamic, the original, and best, comes from Italy. Italian balsamic vinegar is aged in barrels made of ash, cherry, juniper, beech, chestnut, locust, mulberry or white, red or French oak.

18

Authentic balsamic vinegar comes only from Modena, Italy, and begins with grapes. The label on the bottle may say Aceto Balsamico di Modena or Aceto del Duca. In the aging process it is exposed to the heat of Italian summers and the cool of their winters. It is not unusual for a batch to go through as many as a dozen kegs, each made of a different wood. The vinegar's procession from one keg to another is always composed of a succession of both hard and aromatic woods.

19

Never, never taste test pepper vinegar from a spoon - it can be extremely hot and may burn the mouth or tongue. To test hot vinegar, shake a drop or so of this fiery liquid onto a fork full of food and taste the combination.

20

For a special treat, soak meats, fish or poultry in an inexpensive balsamic vinegar before cooking them on the grill. Then, baste the meat frequently with any leftover vinegar.

21

Soak the blossoms of clove pink in champagne vinegar to make a beautiful, delicate pink brew that has a clove-like aroma. Use it as a facial, to deodorized the home or as a perfume that revitalizes the spirit.

22

In medieval times Europeans served foods containing lots of vinegar before and after a feast to aid digestion.

23

A luxury dish of the Roman era was made by cooking apricots in honey, wine and vinegar. Usually, the liquid was thickened and then flavored with pepper and mint.

24

Tradition says that fresh rose petals, added to vinegar, will produce a potion that will inspire love and romance in those who partake of it.

25
Ancient Romans, Greeks and Russians used the aroma of bay leaves to sharpen the memory. Add to vinegar for similar results.

26
Renew the vitality of old vinegar by adding a dash of fresh vinegar to the bottle.

27
Fresh willow twigs, simmered in apple cider vinegar, make a liquid that is great for wiping down boils and skin infections. You can also use it to wet a poultice to apply to a boil.

28
Traditional Chinese Medicine says rue improves mental clarity. European folk medicine calls it an illness preventative. It is a strong herb, so only add one sprig to a pint of vinegar. For super healing, serve this vinegar with garlic and honey mixed with it to make a dressing for greens.

29
French soldiers are reputed to have used vinegar to cool overheated cannons during battles in the 1800s.

30
Romans often preserved turnips by pickling them. Sometimes they were flavored with myrtle berries and honey.

31
Apple cider vinegar is an old folk remedy for arthritis. The traditional way to take it is to mix a teaspoon of vinegar with a teaspoon of clover honey and stir them into a full glass of water. Drink this mixture two or three 3 times a day for relief from the stiffness and pain of arthritis.

February

1

Pamper your skin by bathing in lukewarm water with a couple of cups of strong herbal tea added to it. Make the bath even better for your skin by preparing the tea with apple cider vinegar instead of water.

2

Chinese physicians treat hepatitis with a combination of rice vinegar and B-1 supplements.

3

Greasy pots and pans will clean up easier and require less scrubbing and soap if they are first sprayed with full strength white vinegar. After spraying, let the pans set a few minutes and then wash as usual.

4

Lavender vinegar acts as an effective moth repellant and provides a pleasant aroma in the home.

5

You can use hot pepper vinegar to invigorate your body's metabolism because capsicin, an active compound in hot peppers, is a naturally occurring chemical that can stimulate the body's ability to turn glucose into energy.

6

Pepper vinegar may be safely taste tested by adding a drop of it to a tablespoon of soup.

7

Tabasco® brand hot sauce, most salsas and many curries are made from a base of hot peppers and vinegar.

8

Assure yourself of a blemish-free complexion by regularly patting on a strong onion flavored vinegar. Both the vinegar and the onion juice have antibiotic properties to diminish the possibility of blemishes forming.

9

In the 1500s and 1600s, Europeans cooked thin slices of veal on skews, then served them with vinegar, butter and sugar. It had tangy good taste and covered up the taste of meat that might be slightly spoiled.

10

All food flavors are some combination of sweet, sour, salty or bitter flavors. Vinegar's tartness activates the sour-receptive taste buds along the outside edges of the tongue, because they are the ones most sensitive to the hydrogen ions in its acid. When sweet or salty foods are added to vinegar, they activate other taste receptors that are located on the tip of the tongue. This engagement of the entire mouth in the tasting process results in exceptionally satisfying flavor sensations.

11

2,000 years ago turnips were preserved by pickling them in creamy mustard vinegar. The sauce was made by soaking mustard seeds in water until they were soft, then pounding them into a paste that was mixed with vinegar.

12

As long ago as the time of the ancient Greeks, fennel seeds were popular as an aid to losing weight. Combine fennel's attributes with vinegar by making an herbal dressing to drizzle over foods. To prepare, put 1/2 cup fennel seeds and 2 fresh fennel sprigs into a quart bottle of champagne vinegar and allow to age for three weeks.

13

When balsamic type vinegar is made in the United States it is usually aged in barrels made of bald cypress, basswood, beech, black cherry, elm, red gum, sugar maple, sycamore, white ash or yellow birch barrels.

14

A paste made of oatmeal soaked in apple cider vinegar is said to ease the pain of minor burns.

15

The best vinegar is aged in wood, where its ability to react with its container enhances its flavor.

16

Add oil to vinegar and it is called a vinaigrette (dressing). Add water or juice to vinegar and it becomes a milder, lower calorie alternative to traditional dressings.

17

Vinegar denatures or "cooks" protein. This is called cold cooking and is used for some specialty fish dishes. The customary combination is made with half vinegar and half oil. Any favorite seasonings can be used, too. Use this to "precook" fish to be grilled. Do not soak fish too long or they can "overcook" and dry out. Spices and herbs can make the liquid a more powerful cooking tool.

18

Never store vinegar in metal containers. Its acidic nature reacts with metal and can leach harmful chemicals into the vinegar. It is particularly dangerous to store vinegar in copper, lead or zinc containers.

19

Pour boiling apple cider vinegar over small slivers of slippery elm bark and age for a week. Use this vinegar on a soft cloth to soak the poison from boils and skin infections.

Pepper vinegar that is too hot to use comfortably can be moderated by the addition of extra unseasoned vinegar.

21

Sometimes a small amount of vitamin C may be added to commercially produced vinegar.

22

Wipe dust from the leaves of houseplants with a soft cloth dampened with a mixture of 1/4 cup vinegar and 1 quart water.

23

Vinegar is a wonderfully versatile liquid that can absorb both the flavor and healthful characteristics of herbs and spices. When sprinkled on meats, vegetables and fruits flavored vinegars pass on that goodness.

24

In olden days, olives were preserved by putting them in jars and alternating them with layers of fennel, aromatic resin and vinegar.

25

Drizzle balsamic vinegar over baked beets and serve them with a couple of spoonfuls of sour cream on top.

26

If apples sprayed with the pesticide, Captan, are not thoroughly washed before processing traces of this pesticide can find their way into apple cider vinegar.

27

The double fermentation process by which vinegar is produced predigests the nutrients in the original food used to make it. According to Japanese researchers this makes them much easier for the body to absorb.

28

Moderately priced Italian balsamic vinegar that is intended for export sales is aged for a minimum of seven to ten years. For those who love a great vinegar, and can afford the cost, better grades are aged for 50 years, or even longer.

SPECIAL LEAP YEAR BONUS

For a very special treat, broil new potatoes, slip off their skins, toss with torn spinach and drizzle with a generous amount of balsamic vinegar.

March

1

Make a delicious creamy vinegar-based salad by blending together equal amounts of yogurt and apple cider vinegar. For a spicier dressing, stir in a few tablespoons of brown mustard.

2

Thousands of years enterprising cooks made interesting tasting salads by combining savory, mint, rue, coriander, parsley, chives, lettuce and cheese. These were seasoned with peppered vinegar and a bit of oil.

3

Apple cider vinegar kills bacteria, so rub it into the scalp at bedtime to kill germs that cause itching and flaking.

4

Greasy dishes will clean up with less detergent if 1/4 cup white vinegar is added to the water used to wash them.

5

Stubborn sores and long-lasting skin infections were once treated with external vinegar compresses. Its germ fighting ability was thought to be an aid in healing.

6

A process called "fining" adds chemicals to vinegar to precipitate out any suspended food particles. It makes the product clear and appetizing, but removes nutrients. Bentonite and potassium ferrocyanide casein are sometimes used in fining.

7

Most commercial vinegars are clarified by being filtered, then pasteurized to prevent them from continuing to grow mother after being bottled.

8

Around the lands of the Mediterranean, during the late middle ages, mutton tongue stewed in a mixture of vinegar and orange juice was considered a delicacy.

9

Rice vinegar that has been flavored with ginger and sweetened with brown sugar is used in China to treat allergic itchiness caused by eating fish.

10

Vinegar's complex aroma and taste are mostly due to its rich trace-content of esters and alcohols. Researchers have identified eight different esters and more than a dozen and a half alcohols associated with vinegar.

11

In some European countries a quick process is used to make pseudo balsamic vinegar. Grape juice is heated until it becomes thick and turns brown. Then, it is mixed with ordinary vinegar and wood flavoring. This lesser quality product is used as a substitute for true balsamic vinegar.

12

Traditional Chinese Medicine recommends eating celery that has been cooked in vinegar to relieve a headache that is caused by elevated blood pressure.

13

Use a blender to combine apple cider vinegar and basil leaves to make a creamy vinegar. Sprinkle the ground around tomato plants with this fortified vinegar to keep bugs away.

14

Fennel seeds contain at least 18 different amino acids, 7 minerals (including generous amounts of potassium and calcium) and several vitamins (including lots of vitamin A). Add their good taste and health benefits to your diet by making the following vinegar. Loosely pack a bottle with fennel leaves, add a tablespoon of fennel seeds, fill the bottle with white wine vinegar and cap securely. After three weeks replace the cap with a shaker top and sprinkle it on salads or meats.

15

Asians use good quality vinegar for more than taste. It is an excellent preservative for soy sauce.

16

Old-timers claim that if you dip your hands in apple cider vinegar before working outside in the cold they will not chill as fast as they otherwise would.

17

Traditionally, the ratio of vinegar to oil for making vinaigrettes was one part vinegar to three parts oil. Today's lighter way of eating calls for less oil and lots of herbs for seasoning. Canola, corn, cottonseed, olive, safflower, soybean and sunflower oils are particularly good choices for making vinaigrettes.

18

Large volume, commercially produced vinegars are pasteurized by heating them to about 150°F. If heated above 160°F, flavor and aroma deteriorate.

19

Apple cider vinegar contains small amounts of both calcium and magnesium, two minerals used to boost bone density and fight osteoporosis. Vinegar is also very good at conveying nutrients from one food to another. Just as the chemicals in cayenne peppers and fennel seeds end up in the vinegar in which they are soaked, calcium in chicken bones leaches into vinegar during cooking. This is a good reason to add some vinegar to the water used to boil chicken for soup and other dishes.

20

Mother of vinegar is a living substance and will die if it sinks to the bottom of the fermenting liquid and loses its air supply. Jolting the container of brewing vinegar can cause this to happen. Often a sliver of wood, slice of bread or corn cob serves as a raft to help the mother to remain floating on the surface.

21

The very best balsamic vinegar is not usually available outside the Modena area of Italy, when it is aged more than 75 years.

22

Vinegar, when combined with spicy foods such as horseradish, hot mustard and red pepper, acts as a decongestant.

23

In the days when stuffed suckling pig was the main dish for a banquet it was often basted with lard and vinegar before being roasted. Then, it was eaten with bread crumbs boiled with vinegar, ginger, saffron and cloves.

24

When Roman soldiers went marching off to war, they took along large supplies of vinegar to mix with the local water. Adding vinegar to local water helped to kill bacteria and also masked any unusual taste.

25

Cover small onions with water and boil until tender. Place in a baking dish and sprinkle on four tablespoons of brown sugar and two tablespoons of balsamic vinegar. Bake, uncovered, until sugar is caramelized.

26

Built up water scale on shower heads can be dissolved by soaking the showerhead in white vinegar. Simply wrap paper towels saturated with white vinegar around the showerhead. Cover with a plastic bag, secure with a rubber band and let set overnight. The next morning, brush the showerhead with additional vinegar and the scale will melt away.

27

To make a delicious, intensely flavored vinaigrette mix 1/2 cup apple cider vinegar and 1/2 cup oil with 1/4 teaspoon each of basil, minced garlic, oregano, parsley, tarragon and thyme.

28

Vinegar's acid does more than simply add flavor to food; it also softens tough fibers. To make an excellent tenderizing marinade, begin with 1/2 cup apple cider vinegar and 1/2 cup oil. Next, add sliced lemon, bay leaves, thyme, paprika or other spices and herbs. Use this to marinate foods before broiling or grilling and it will shorten the cooking time while it improves flavors.

29

When vinegar and baking soda are combined they provide leavening for baked goods by creating bubbles of carbon dioxide and water. Then, as the baking process continues, these small droplets of water turn into steam. Each droplet of water expands to 1600 times its original size when it becomes steam. Because the steam is contained within the baked goods, this moisture has tremendous power to leaven the baked goods.

30

Even heavy pie crust dough can use the terrific power of carbon dioxide based steam for leavening. The following recipe for vinegar pastry makes enough dough for a double crust pie. Sift together 1 cup flour and 1/2 teaspoon baking powder. Add 1/4 cup oil, 1 egg white, 3 tablespoons vinegar, 3 tablespoons water, 1 tablespoon sugar and 1/2 teaspoon salt (optional). Mix all ingredients together with a fork and roll out.

31

Refined Europeans of the 1600s and 1700s carried little boxes, called vinaigrettes, as holders for vinegar soaked sponges. Tiny openings in the tops allowed them to sniff the vinegar to protect themselves from the foul odors and diseases that plagued city life. Often these boxes were made of gold or silver.

April

1

When varnished wood comes in contact with water it can develop a hazy surface. Prevent this by adding a teaspoon of white vinegar to each cup of water used to wash wood; then immediately dry the surface.

2

Sometimes Modena vinegar, the king of balsamic vinegars, is simply sipped as an after dinner treat.

3

The enzymes in vinegar, one of the by-products of its fermentation process, make other foods more digestible. For example, vinegar's carbohydrate is 98% digestible.

4

To remove musty odors from a glass jar, dampen a sponge with a teaspoon or two of white vinegar and close it in the jar for at least 30 minutes. It will smell fresh and clean again.

5

Fruit flavored vinegars were used to flavor drinks in the 1700s and 1800s, much as lemons are used to make lemonade today.

6

Researchers at the Chinese Academy of Medical Science report that the vapors of boiling vinegar can kill the germs that cause pneumonia and also those that cause influenza.

7

Preserve home-made vinegar in small bottles, filled to the top, to minimize the amount of air exposure. This will help retain its full flavor and strength.

8

Keep your pets' water dishes clean and odor free by soaking them for 20 minutes a day in vinegar. This will discourage bacteria from growing on these perpetually wet surfaces. And, it avoids the need to use chlorine disinfectants (such as bleach) that may be harmful to the animal.

9

Clean and brighten most kinds of wood paneling by wiping them down with a solution made of 1 cup warm water, 1 tablespoon white vinegar and 1 tablespoon olive oil. Be sure to mix well and use immediately. Dry the paneling with a soft, clean cloth.

10

Two tablespoons of ginger vinegar, stirred into a glass of water and sipped slowly is said to relieve a digestive system that has been stressed by eating too much fruit.

11

If you add a splash of apple cider vinegar to a horse's water each day its coat will lose any dullness and develop a healthy shine. A little vinegar each day will also perk up a horse's sluggish appetite.

12

Aphids will be reluctant to attack cabbage, Brussel sprouts and cauliflower plants if you wet a circle of ground around them with mint vinegar.

13

Enzymes in vinegar influence the body's rate of metabolism. Metabolism moderates chemical changes in the cells that provide energy to the body. This includes the way fats are burned.

14

Freshen and deodorize any room by setting a bowl of hot water with a cup of apple cider vinegar and a dash of cinnamon in it on a low table.

15

Blend 1/2 cup apple cider vinegar, 1/2 cup orange juice and 2 table-spoons mustard to make a mild dressing for mixed greens.

16

In the late middle ages, in the large manor houses of Europe's feudal estates, carrots were frequently cooked with honey and vinegar.

17

Apple cider vinegar is good for chickens of all ages. Peeps will be bigger and healthier if a bit of apple cider vinegar is added to their drinking water. And later, it will strengthen the shells of their eggs.

18

A fortified vinegar is one that has had tiny pieces of fruit or vegetables blended into it. Apple fortified vinegar is a good way to fight cancer, because it increases the amount of fiber in the diet. It also adds important amino acids to strengthen the immune system in its battle against all types of disease.

19

After shampooing, rinse the hair with an herbal fortified vinegar to rid the hair of soap traces. This will also give it a fresh scent and help to discourage the development of dandruff.

20

With advancing age, sometimes the stomach does not produce the amount of acid needed for good digestion. Perhaps this is why vinegar has long been considered a digestive aid.

21

To preserve garlic cloves, simply peel and cover with vinegar. CAUTION: Never store garlic in oil - without the addition of vinegar. Garlic preserved in only oil can result in botulism tainted oil. (Botulism cannot be detected by odor or taste.)

22

Vinegar that has not been distilled has more particles of its original food in it than vinegar that has been distilled. This is one good reason to use organic vinegar that has been processed as little as possible.

23

Vinegar that has had fennel seeds soaked in it is considered by many to be an aid to good digestion. Medical research indicates that fennel seeds contain substances that react to fats. In addition, they contain a hormone-like substance, which may explain why they are recommended in old-time remedies for helping nursing mothers to increase the amount of milk they produce.

24

A paste of wood ashes and vinegar was used by the Greeks of olden times to treat skin eruptions.

25

Including flowers in scented vinegars can add to vinegar's natural astringent qualities. Spices and herbs do this, too. Because vinegar's pH is almost the same as that of healthy skin, it soothes and normalizes its surface.

26

2,000 years ago a banquet might feature pork shoulder cooked with tenderizing vinegar. Tender morsels of this popular meat were then served in a sauce of apricots, honey and wine, seasoned with pepper and mint.

27

Mix 1/4 cup garlic flavored apple cider vinegar with 1/4 cup water and 1/2 teaspoon honey to make a gentle vinaigrette that softens vinegar's usual tartness.

28

When vinegar is aged in wooden barrels its flavor "ripens" and becomes mellow. Over many years it develops sophisticated esters and ethers that contribute to a more complicated taste than ordinary vinegar.

29

Vinegar moderates the oily taste of fried foods such as fish and French fries. Keep it in a spray bottle and mist these foods just before serving to leave a clear, less greasy taste in the mouth.

30

The British spray straight malt vinegar on deep fried potatoes. Americans are more likely to douse fries with apple cider vinegar flavored with tomato sauce (a condiment called catsup).

May

1

In the lands around the Mediterranean, in ancient days, a feast was often begun with a dish of chopped olives. They were mixed with vinegar, oil and spices such as coriander, cumin, fennel, rue and mint.

2

Ancient Romans safely ate oysters because they served them in a vinegar-based sauce that helped preserve them.

3

In Traditional Chinese Medicine herbs are often processed in vinegar to increase their effectiveness.

4

Never heat pretty herbal vinegar in an iron pan. The metal may cause the vinegar to turn very dark, even black, as it leaches iron from the pan.

5

An old-time remedy for a sluggish appetite is to nibble on small bits of meat that has been cooked with a generous dash of vinegar.

6

For more than 2,000 years Asians have used ginger, soaked in vinegar, to prevent and relieve motion sickness and other digestive upsets.

7

In Old Testament Bible times most meals included a bowl of honey (called oxybaphon) and a bowl of vinegar (called acetabulum) to dip bread into. These common dipping bowls were part of everyday life, as evidenced by Boaz's invitation to Ruth to share his table and communal vinegar bowl. This tradition extended well into New Testament times.

8

Tarragon vinegar, when it ages, oxidizes into a brew that tastes very much like dill flavored vinegar.

9

Greeks, as well as Asians, have long considered plums preserved in vinegar to be a special delicacy.

10

For many thousands of years, doctors in China have treated the symptoms of food poisoning from contaminated fish, meat or vegetables by having the affected person sip on rice vinegar.

11

Vinegar's healing ways have long been used to both prevent and fight disease. Japanese scientists have shown that vinegar kills germs that can cause colitis, dysentery and some of the most common forms of food poisoning.

12

For an old-time delicacy, clean the seeds out of hot peppers and broil them until they begin to brown. Immediately sprinkle them with balsamic vinegar and enjoy!

13

Freshen stale smelling plasticware containers by putting a paper towel moistened with vinegar in it. Seal up the container and allow to set overnight. By morning the offending odor will have disappeared.

14

Ancient civilizations put much faith in the healthfulness of food combinations that brought sweet and sour tastes together in the same dish. You can prepare a dish that combines ancient faith with today's taste in foods by seasoning greens with a creamy honey-mustard salad dressing. Simply combine 1/4 cup sweet clover honey, 1/4 cup tart apple cider vinegar and 1 tablespoon spicy yellow mustard.

15

Mosquitoes will avoid your yard if it is sprinkled occasionally with diluted lavender vinegar.

16

An old adage says you can ease the pain of a toothache by holding a mix of vinegar and water in the mouth for a minute or so. Dentists today would NOT recommend this!

17

By the 1700s, people in England used vinegar as a healing gargle, much as we do today.

18

Vinegar which has had salted hot peppers soaked in it is sometimes called 'liquid pepper.' (If you have tasted it, you know why.)

19

In the ancient world, vinegar was considered the treatment of choice for those who had eaten poisonous mushrooms.

20

This chocolate-vinegar cake uses vinegar to replace the leavening sometimes supplied by eggs. Combine 1 cup brown sugar, 2 tablespoons cocoa, 1/4 cup oil, 1 teaspoon baking soda, 1 teaspoon vanilla, 1 cup milk, 2 teaspoons vinegar, 1 1/2 cups flour, 1/4 teaspoon baking powder and 1/4 teaspoon salt. Bake at 350°F. for about 30 minutes.

21

To make a rich vinaigrette for drizzling over greens, combine 1/4 cup red wine vinegar and 3/4 cup oil, then add a teaspoon each of coarse salt and freshly ground black pepper.

22

An old-time favorite for easing coughs is a syrup made of baked and mashed garlic, honey and apple cider vinegar.

23

To ease indigestion after eating fish, an old-time home remedy is to sip on water with a tablespoon or so of ginger vinegar added to it. Make this healing vinegar by grating a teaspoon of fresh ginger root into two cups of rice vinegar and allowing it to sit for at least a week before using.

24

In Australia, vinegar is regularly sprayed on raw meat to slow the action of the bacteria which causes it to rot.

25

Pectin is a water soluble fiber that is plentiful in apples. It slows the absorption of food in the intestines, allowing it to bind to cholesterol. Make a cholesterol fighting, fortified vinegar by combining 2 cups chopped apples, 1 cup apple cider vinegar and 1/2 cup honey in a blender. Season with 1/2 teaspoon cinnamon and 1/4 teaspoon nutmeg and serve over fruit salad.

26

A very old balsamic vinegar can cost more than a hundred dollars for a small bottle. One reason is that as vinegar is moved from one wooden barrel to another during the aging process there is less and less vinegar as it becomes concentrated.

27

Asians have long claimed that substances in the ginkgo plant can improve the mind. To make vinegar enhanced with ginkgo's goodness, place fresh leaves in a bottle and cover them with vinegar. Let set for at least two weeks before using.

28

Prepare a delightful fruit salad dressing by combining 1 cup apple cider vinegar, 2 cups raspberries and 1/2 cup mint leaves in a blender. Pour this sauce over fresh mixed fruit or drizzle several spoonfuls over a slice of ripe melon.

29

Test the aroma of a great balsamic vinegar by pouring a small amount into a short, wide glass. Then, swirl the liquid and delicately sniff the aroma from a few inches above the glass.

30

Folklore claims that the regular addition of vinegar to the diet will enhance the health of both the liver and the stomach.

31

Hot pepper vinegar can be a self-defense food that is effective for personal protection. A good splash of this fiery liquid on the face or in the eyes should send an attacker running

June

1

Vinegar that has had oregano leaves soaked in it makes a good barricade against insects that gather on cucumbers. Wet the ground around young plants once a week. This will also help keep bugs from eating the leaves of melon plants.

2

For a healthy vegetable treat, steam stalks of asparagus and celery until they are barely tender, then drizzle them with fennel flavored vinegar and garnish with fresh parsley.

3

Ancient Greeks sliced turnips very thin, dusted them with salt, then soaked them in vinegar. These pickled turnips were often flavored with mustard seeds and raisins.

4

In Colonial times fevers were often treated by wiping the entire body down with full strength apple cider vinegar.

5

Use white vinegar in the water when rinsing wool sweaters and they will be fluffier than if rinsed in plain water.

6

Prevent apples for pie from turning brown by slicing them into a bowl of water with 1/4 cup white vinegar added to it. Drain the water and vinegar off of the apples before cooking.

7

Set dishes of lavender vinegar around your kitchen and flies will not be a problem. It is also helpful to spray it on and around your picnic table.

8

After bathing a long-haired cat, rinse it with a quart of water with three or four tablespoons of vinegar added to it. This will make the fur shine and tangles will brush out much easier.

9

Hippocrates suggested easing troubled breathing with a mixture of vinegar, honey and garlic. One way to make this beneficial syrup is to simmer peeled garlic cloves in enough apple cider vinegar to cover them. When the cloves are soft, mash them into the vinegar and add a spoonful of honey to the mixture.

10

Watercress, soaked in vinegar, was used by the Romans of long ago to treat those with mental problems.

11

Comparing the taste of one vinegar to another is not easy because vinegar is so acidic that, at the first sip, the taste buds shut down. This makes it very difficult to accurately taste test a second sample. This natural reaction can be minimized by sampling vinegar on a sugar cube. Dip the sugar into the vinegar and taste test the flavored cube.

12

Reactivate the taste buds between tasting different vinegars by sipping a bit of seltzer water. Or, try nibbling on unsalted crackers; they will help to reset the taste buds.

13

Kill grass and weeds that sprout in your driveway or in sidewalk cracks by drenching them with vinegar.

14

Molds, yeasts and bacteria are essential to life, but they can cause problems when they attack food. Meat is particularly susceptible to contamination by nasty microorganisms. If vinegar is sprayed on beef, it dramatically reduces the number of germs. And, its action lasts more than a week! This procedure is also effective on pork.

15

Baked goods that contain vinegar stay fresh and editable longer than those without it because they are much slower to produce mold.

16

Prevent water-borne infections from settling in the ears by rinsing them out with a mixture of 1/2 rubbing alcohol and 1/2 vinegar.

17

A healthy substitute for popular sports drinks can be easily made from vinegar. Simply fill a glass half way with crushed ice and add 4 to 6 drops of a good quality balsamic vinegar. Fill the glass with cold water and swirl. Sip slowly.

18

In Italy, balsamic vinegar can still be found aging in casks that date from the 1700s.

19

The very best balsamic vinegar is so prized in some regions of Italy that it is apt to be part of a young lady's dowry.

20

Garden lime and other corrosive alkali based products can cause chemical burns on cats. If your cat is exposed to any of these poisons, thoroughly rinse the cat with a mixture of one quart vinegar and one quart water. Repeat as necessary.

21

You can zip up the taste of homemade soups with a dash of any zesty herbal vinegar. Add the vinegar just before serving to keep the herbal aroma fresh. You may also want to put the vinegar on the table so that more adventurous folks can add even more vinegar to their bowls.

22

Balsamic vinegar can be expensive, but you can make your own good imitation by mixing concentrated frozen grape juice and brown sugar with apple cider vinegar.

23

Because vinegar was one of the first ways discovered to protect food from bacterial attack, it developed an early reputation as a wondrous, nearly mystic substance. Even highly perishable foods, such as meats, seafood and eggs were preserved in vinegar.

24

Sprinkle fennel vinegar around the stall of an unruly cow or horse and it will calm them down and improve their disposition.

25

Historically, both the Greeks and the Romans imported large quantities of vinegar from Egypt. Egyptian vinegar was considered one of the most excellent varieties in the ancient world.

26

Scientists believe vinegar had an important role in the creation of life. They tell us it was part of the primordial soup that provided a chemical start for life, because when vinegar is combined with ammonia, it makes up the simplest biologically important building block of life!

27

Vinegar can be an important part of delicious desserts. One mouth-watering treat can be made by dribbling a teaspoon of fortified fruit vinegar over vanilla ice cream. Add slivers of dark chocolate and then top it all with a sprinkling of raw sugar.

28

To make a sweet raspberry vinegar, bring 2 cups sugar and 1 cup water to a boil. Add 2 cups fresh or frozen raspberries and simmer until the fruit is tender (about 1 minute). Add this to 1 quart vinegar, refrigerate and allow to sit for 24 hours. Strain, then add a dozen firm, just barely ripe berries to the bottle.

29

When vinegar is made from bananas, they are mashed for the first fermentation, then the chunks are filtered out before the second fermentation.

30

Vinegar producers of the 1800s found they could make acetic acid from wood chips, or even from the residues discarded during paper making. These companies added flavorings and color and called the result apple cider vinegar. This cheap imitation was, of course, deficient in taste and aroma, and did not contain the vast array of natural enzymes and nutrients of the original. Today's labeling laws prevent this kind of product adulteration - if the bottle says apple cider vinegar - it contains vinegar that began life as apples.

July

1

Add zest to ordinary mayonnaise by adding a teaspoon of apple cider vinegar to each four tablespoons of mayonnaise. Use this spread for hot weather sandwiches to help prevent food poisoning. (Vinegar is the main preservative in catsup, mayonnaise, pickles and most salad dressings.) for a more intense flavor, use an herbal or fortified vinegar.

2

Are your carpets beginning to look dreary and dull? Or have they developed unpleasant odors? Brighten and deodorize them by spraying on a cleaning liquid made of 1 cup white vinegar to a gallon of water. Immediately wipe the spray off with a soft, absorbent cloth. Colors will seem to glow and musky odors will fade away. (Always, always test your carpet first!)

3

Spray picnic tables with bay flavored apple cider vinegar to keep flies from settling on food. It will also make the air smell fresh and pleasant, while stimulating appetites.

4

Fennel vinegar is an excellent topping for broiled fish. Make your own by soaking fennel seeds in apple cider vinegar.

5

Some researchers have reported that hot pepper vinegar's naturally occurring cayenne contains a substance that is able to stimulate the brain's pleasure-sensitive endorphins.

6

Add a cup of white vinegar to washing machine rinse water and cotton blankets will be softer and smell fresh longer than if rinsed without this natural odor and soap scum remover.

7

Sprinkle a strong infusion of rue vinegar around doorways to discourage fleas from entering your house.

8

A very strong thyme vinegar makes a great pest repellent! Use it on garden paths and on patio stones to keep creeping and flying insects away. It will also leave a pleasant odor in the air.

9

Pickle boiled beets by submerging them in 1 cup apple cider vinegar mixed with 1/2 cup water and 1/4 cup sugar. Add pepper and mustard to taste.

10

For an easy, delightful tasting treat, drizzle sweet raspberry vinegar over mixed greens that have been sprinkled with grated hazelnuts.

11

When slicing peaches for canning, keep them in a bath of water with a dash of white vinegar added to it and they will not turn brown. (Drain well before canning.)

12

Soak the area where pets spend their time with vinegar that has been enhanced with fennel; it will discourage fleas from congregating. Rue vinegar will also discourage fleas. Rub it into a dog or cat's fur and use it to wipe down the outside of feeding dishes.

13

To reduce calories and increase good taste, replace high calorie gravy with strained meat juice, sharpened with a splash of vinegar and seasoned with your favorite herbs.

14

In ancient times raw cabbage was dipped in vinegar because it was thought to make it as digestible as if it were cooked.

15

Bacteria on meat can cause it to change color as it reacts with air. Vinegar sprayed on meat slows this color change. This is very important to retailers, because many customers judge meat's freshness and quality by its color.

16

Brown rice vinegar is sweeter than white rice vinegar and more expensive. This vinegar is used in soy sauces and is good on stir-fried foods, especially noodles.

17

An old-time liniment for relieving the aches and pains of arthritis and rheumatism is made by combining hot peppers and vinegar. Recently, medical researchers have confirmed the usefulness of this pain reliever.

18

The capsicin that makes peppers hot has been proven by researchers to interfere with the way nerve endings in the skin send pain messages to the brain. This is one reason why old-fashioned folk remedies for arthritis and rheumatism often used vinegar that had hot peppers in it worked so well to relieve muscle and joint pain.

19

Spray basil vinegar around doors and windows to discourage flies from entering your home.

20

Vinegar is the cleaner of choice for those who have allergies. Its fresh odor is much less likely to cause sneezing or itching than harsh chemical cleaners.

21

Use lusty red wine vinegar with strong herbs, white wine vinegar with more gentle ones. Champagne vinegar is an excellent base for berry or delicate herb mixtures. Sherry vinegar goes well with nutty flavors.

Use vinegar in the kitchen to sanitize cutting boards and other surfaces touched by raw meats. Simply wipe surfaces down with full strength white or apple cider vinegar.

23

A creamy fortified garlic vinegar adds vitamins to the diet. Medical research shows a multivitamin enriched diet can activate the immune system. For a creamy garlic vinegar, boil half a cup of peeled garlic cloves in just enough water to cover them. When the garlic is soft, mix them in a blender with an equal amount of apple cider vinegar. For a more tart dressing add more vinegar; for a less tart dressing add a small amount of water.

24

Prepare a smooth, creamy vinaigrette by blending 1/4 cup each of vinegar, oil and yogurt. Use immediately. This dressing is especially good when seasoned with a tablespoon of parsley or chives (or both).

25

For a salad dressing with a nice sweet-sour combination combine 1/4 cup apple cider vinegar, 1 teaspoon honey and 1/4 teaspoon paprika. Give your dressing extra zip and restorative power by substituting hot pepper vinegar. This is also a great low calorie topping for boiled vegetables.

26

Vinegar can be a great help to anyone on a reduced salt diet. The unique, zesty tartness of vinegar helps reduce the amount of salt needed to flavor food.

27

If your cat leaves a urine stain on your carpet, lift the stain by blotting up as much of the liquid as possible, then sprinkling the area with white vinegar. Blot until the carpet is dry and repeat as necessary. (Always test carpet before using ANY cleaning substance on it, even one as mild as vinegar.)

28

The cayenne that gives hot pepper vinegar its zing has been shown to stabilize blood pressure. Only a very small amount is necessary to achieve this benefit.

29

Garlic, such as that in creamy fortified vinegars, can lower both cholesterol and blood pressure. This marvelous combination also contains chemicals researchers have found to be able to improve memory and increase the ability to learn in old age.

30

It was once thought that serving beet leaves, lentils and beans in a vinegar dressing would strengthen the digestive system.

31

Never store vinegar for salads in a cruet with a high lead content. Lead crystal, over time, can leach poisonous lead into vinegar.

August

1

The exact chemical content of vinegar depends on the kind of food used to make it. For example, apple cider vinegar is the only kind of vinegar that contains malic acid.

2

Vinegar added to the sugar for making taffy helps turn the sucrose of white sugar into glucose and fructose. This inversion process is what makes the length of cooking time critical. If the syrup is not cooked long enough, there will be insufficient invert sugar, and so the candy will be gritty. If the syrup is cooked too long, too much of the sugar will become invert and there will not be enough sucrose left to crystallize and so the candy will be too soft.

3

Make old-fashioned pulled taffy by combining 2 cups sugar, 2/3 cup water and 1 tablespoon vinegar in a good sized saucepan. Stir while the mixture heats, but not after it comes to a boil. Cook to the hardball stage for a chewy candy, to the soft crack stage for a more brittle candy. Remove from heat, swirl in 1 teaspoon butter and 1/2 teaspoon vanilla and pour onto a cool, buttered (or oiled) surface. As it becomes cool enough to handle, work the mixture until it changes color and begins to set up. Then, quickly cut it into bite-sized pieces.

4

Spatter small droplets of a robust sage vinegar on the ground near vegetable vines to keep harmful insects from attacking your garden plants.

5

Often, stains can be lifted from permanent press fabrics by wetting the stain with white vinegar, letting it set for a few minutes, then washing with detergent and cool water.

6

Over the years, some vinegar makers have added sulphites to their product to extend its shelf life. Others have added salt. Read vinegar labels carefully to avoid these additives.

7

In the writings of Pliny, an ancient Roman poet, we are told of his liking for lettuce served with a mustard seed and vinegar sauce. He also recommended cooking the large, coarse leaves of elecampane in vinegar before drying it (we call this sunflower look-alike sneeze weed or horseheal).

8

Always protect pearls from contact with vinegar. Prolonged contact can damage them and, eventually, completely dissolve them.

9

Wipe down dogs and cats coats with apple cider vinegar that has had camomile flowers soaked in it to discourage ticks from bothering them. Dabbing their fur with it will also help to repel fleas.

10

Surprisingly, the cayenne in hot pepper vinegar does not seem to irritate ulcers.

11

To make a clear, super-hot pepper vinegar, pack a jar with tiny cayenne peppers. Leave half of them whole and cut the remaining peppers in half, lengthways. (Include or substitute other hot peppers, such as jalapenos if you wish.) Cover with vinegar and age for 3 weeks. As the liquid is used, add additional vinegar for a continuing supply of intense flavoring.

12

Vinegar is an antimicrobial agent, effective against yeasts, bacteria and molds. This makes it a good germ fighter in the kitchen.

13

Vinegar (acetic acid) is present in most plant and animal tissues. Even the human body makes some. It is needed to burn both fats and carbohydrates. It also plays a role in how the body stores fat. When vinegar enters the blood stream it is carried to the kidneys and muscles. There, it is either oxidized into pure energy or used to make body tissues, through its ability to make essential amino acids. It even facilitates the process that forms the red blood cells that supply the body's oxygen.

14

After washing greasy kitchen exhaust fans and air conditioner grills, wipe the exposed surfaces down with white vinegar. This will retard a future buildup of grease and dust and leave your kitchen smelling fresh and clean.

15

Wet the foundation of your home with a very strong infusion of mint vinegar to protect it from rats.

16

Herbal vinegar made by putting wintergreen clippings in warm apple cider vinegar is reputed to ease muscle aches when it is rubbed into them.

17

You can combine the 10,000 phytochemicals in tomatoes with the super healing powers of hot peppers and vinegar by making salsa. Chop 1/2 cup chilies, 1 cup tomatoes and 1 cup onions. Mix all the chopped vegetables together and add 1 teaspoon sugar and 1/2 cup vinegar. Let the mixture set overnight so that the assortment of flavors have time to blend. Use this healthy salsa as a dip for corn flour based chips or pile it on rice cakes for an interesting mix of low calorie tastes. (Optional ingredients: salt, black pepper and garlic.)

18

Rid the kitchen of the smell of scorched or burnt food by spritzing the air with vinegar. Either white, apple cider or herbal vinegar work well.

19

Patent leather shoes will gleam like new if you wipe them down with a paper towel moistened with full strength white vinegar. After cleaning them with vinegar, preserve them by applying a thin coating of petroleum jelly and then buffing them with a soft cloth.

20

Vinegar is effective in killing salmonella and staphylococcus, as well as at least five other germs.

21

Intensify the goodness of any ginger flavored dish by added a dash of hot pepper vinegar. This is a good way to add zip to ginger ale, too. Try stirring in a spoonful of hot pepper vinegar and be prepared for a treat.

22

A garlic fortified vinegar, made by combining lots of cooked garlic cloves and vinegar in a blender is an extremely healthy way to add flavor to bland vegetables.

23

Steep new leaves of the lavender plant in vinegar for 10 days, then strain them out and use the vinegar as a wash for the inside of storage areas for clothes. It will drive away moths and leave a pleasant aroma in these dark areas.

24

Always use hot pepper vinegar with great caution. Both hot peppers and the vinegar that they have been steeped in can burn the sensitive lining of the mouth and tongue and blister skin.

25

If ripe olives are soaked in vinegar for a few hours it will be much easier to remove their pits.

26

Vinegar compresses have been used for hundreds of years as an effective and safe way to disinfect sores on horses. It is also safe for treating minor scraps and abrasions on dogs and goats.

27

The acid that we know as vinegar is used by the body as a detoxifying agent. Molecules of this amazing liquid are able to connect themselves to many dangerous substances, including some drugs and poisons. This action creates entirely new compounds, which tend to be biologically inactive. Then, these harmless substances can be safely expelled by the body.

28

Rich Romans served endive with vinegar and honey. This was especially welcome during wintertime when other greens were less available.

29

Put a little vinegar in the water you use to cook beans, cabbage or broccoli to reduce the amount of gas producing chemicals in these foods.

30

When housecleaning, add vinegar to rinse water and it will prevent soap scum from dulling painted surfaces, vinyl floors, countertops and appliances.

31

For thousands of years vinegar was used as a universal remedy for poisoning because it was thought to neutralize them.

September

1

A vinegar tonic before meals has long been recommended to help those with low stomach acid digest food more thoroughly so they can pull more nutrients form their food.

2

Vinegar is both antiseptic and antibiotic; it also neutralizes alkali burns.

3

Researchers have found that an ingredient in hot pepper vinegar is able to moderate excessive bleeding.

4

Old-timers believe that the capsicin released from hot peppers when they were soaked in vinegar could work as an internal remedy for the aches of arthritis and rheumatism.

5

In the days when the Roman Empire flourished, vinegar and salt were used to pickle asparagus.

6

Clothes which have been exposed to cigarette or cigar smoke can be deodorized by hanging them over a bathtub containing two cups of apple cider vinegar added to some very hot water.

7

To make a fiery hot vinegar, combine a dozen cayennes in a blender with 1 cup apple cider vinegar. Make it even better by adding 5 peeled garlic cloves and 2 medium onions. Use this sizzling vinegar with caution.

8

Pour full-strength vinegar over fire ant hills to drive them away from your property. Spray vinegar in cupboards to discourage ants in the house.

9

Very old, concentrated, balsamic vinegars are mild and mellow enough to be used as a complete dressing, without the addition of oil or spices. Younger vinegars are not as smooth.

10

Old timers promised fewer bladder infections for those who took a vinegar tonic every day. It was said that this practice would produce urine with a higher acid content, to discourage bacteria infections.

11

White vinegar is the least expensive variety, so is a good choice for cleaning. It is also less likely to stain because it has been filtered so that it contains few trace elements from the originating product that might react with surfaces to be cleaned.

12

In a pinch, use vinegar as a substitute deodorant. Try it on underarms and feet.

13

Sipping on rice vinegar was used by Traditional Chinese Medicine to ease the vomiting of blood. It was also considered helpful to those suffering from nosebleeds.

14

According to Traditional Chinese Medicine peanuts soaked overnight in vinegar can lower blood pressure. These Chinese practitioners recommend eating several of the pickled nuts each day for 2 weeks.

15

Boiled rice will be snowy white and extra fluffy if a tablespoon of white vinegar is added to the water in which it is cooked.

16

A little vinegar added to the water used for boiling cabbage will keep your kitchen from smelling of cooked cabbage.

17

If pickles are too sour, soften the intensity of their taste by stirring in some sugar 1 hour before serving. Or, drain off 1/2 of the liquid covering them and replace it with water. Allow to set overnight, refrigerated, before serving. Make pickles extra-sour by draining off 3/4 of their liquid and replacing it with new vinegar.

18

Use herbal vinegars to add unique tastes, not calories, to your weight loss diet. Dash it onto cooked or raw veggies and fruits or on to broiled fish.

19

Do not store foods enhanced with vinegar in old bread wrappers or plastic bags with advertising on them. Unpleasant chemicals in printed material may be pulled into the food.

20

All vinegar is not created equal. Its aroma and flavor are influenced by the way it is made and aged. Vinegar is a complex substance, brimming with subtle flavors and aromas and packed with an assortment of nutrients, enzymes and trace elements. The best vinegar is a combination of sweet mellowness from wooden storage barrels and the sharp, sour zing of acetic acid.

Since ancient times fennel has been used to aid digestion and add vitamins A and C, calcium, phosphorus and potassium to the diet. Combining a cup of tightly packed fennel leaves and half a cup of champagne vinegar in a blender results in an excellent salad dressing. To make it even better, add a teaspoon of fennel seeds and six peppercorns to the mixture.

22

Freshen up a stale smelling camper by spritzing walls, countertops and floors with white vinegar. Air old foam mattresses in the sun, after spraying them lightly, too.

23

Perk up the taste of melon slices by sprinkling them with honey-sweetened thyme vinegar.

24

Soak sprigs of fresh wintergreen in apple cider vinegar for two weeks. The resulting herbal vinegar makes a great skin softener that can be useful on calluses.

25

Submerge freshly picked leafy greens in water that has had a small dash of salt and a large splash of vinegar added to it. Any bugs hiding in the greens will float to the top of the water.

26

Jellyfish stings can be deadly to dogs. Immediately pour lots of full strength vinegar over a sting to neutralize the poison.

27

Try a fortified vinegar today! Their thick, creamy goodness is an especially pleasant way to add health promoting fruits and vegetables to your diet.

28

Paris street markets, in the 1700s, offered more than 50 kinds of flavored cooking vinegars. And, more than 90 varieties were to be found for making the outside of the body smell better. The most popular, and least expensive, was pepper vinegar. It was made from wine that had been laced with pepper. Other common vinegar flavors of that day included: clove, carnation, chicory, mustard, fennel, ginger, pistachio, rose and truffle.

29

Vinegar has almost exactly the same pH rating as healthy human skin. This is why it is such a healing balm for distressed skin.

30

Add vinegar to the rinse water in your washing machine and colored clothes will stay brighter, longer.

October

1

If you pet sprains a leg muscle, wrap it in strips cut from a brown paper bag that has been soaked in apple cider vinegar. The animal will feel better faster.

2

When soap scum and hard water minerals build up on drinking glasses, vases, mixing bowls, cups, etc., it makes them look old and dull. A good soaking in full strength white vinegar will dissolve the hazy film and bring back their natural, clear beauty.

3

Vinegar folklore promised that the intense pain of shingles could be moderated by eating food that was well-laced with hot pepper vinegar. Supposedly, the capsicin the peppers released into the vinegar was the soothing agent.

4

Clean and freshen ashtrays by wiping them out with either apple cider or white vinegar, diluted half and half with warm water. If badly stained, soak them with full strength vinegar.

5

Folklore has long promised that nibbling on mother of vinegar will energize your immune system.

6

Soak canned shrimp in equal parts water and vinegar to perk up the flavor and freshen their taste.

7

Apple cider vinegar, laced with lots of fennel seeds, makes a toping for foods that is not only tasty but contains health-promoting flavonoids.

8

In addition to the alkaloid called capsaicin, cayenne peppers add vitamins A and C, flavonoids and carotenoids to vinegar's normal inventory of beneficial ingredients.

9

Vinegar's history is as old as that of mankind. The first vinegar probably began as wine that was exposed to air. Wild yeasts fermented it into a wonderful, life-enhancing liquid!

10

Because it could be stored for months, pickled cabbage was popular in Poland and Hungary during the 1700s. Today, it is more popular served as a freshly vinegared vegetable. One low calorie way to do this is to make coleslaw. Begin by shredding 3 cups cabbage and 1/2 cup carrots. Sprinkle the vegetables with 1/4 cup sugar, cover with cold water and add a tight fitting lid. Set aside for 2 hours and then drain off all of the liquid. Dress with champagne vinegar diluted half and half with water.

11

Kill germs and deter mold and fungus growth in garages by spraying surfaces liberally with vinegar.

12

In Italy, balsamic vinegar sprinkled on fresh strawberries is considered a special dessert delicacy. Because of balsamic vinegar's mild nature and concentrated good flavor it is good on fruit, with no need for the addition of sugar or spices.

13

Eating foods seasoned with hot pepper vinegar encourages the body to produce natural anti-inflammatory chemicals.

14

Old-fashioned ladies got rid of facial blemishes by applying a paste of corn starch, honey and vinegar.

15

True balsamic vinegar, from the Modena region of Italy, is often aged in wooden barrels for 50 years – or longer!

16

You can make a calcium-rich soup stock by beginning with a whole, cut up chicken. Cover it with water, add 1/2 cup herb flavored vinegar and gently simmer for 2 hours. The herbs will add subtle flavor to your stock and the vinegar will leach calcium from the chicken's bones. Use this stock to make calcium-enriched casseroles and gravies.

17

When preparing vinaigrettes, combine vinegar with healthy oils, such as olive, safflower or sunflower.

18

For great tasting boiled hot dogs add a generous splash of apple cider vinegar to the water they are boiled in.

19

Keep the skin healthy by spraying your body with a dilute vinegar and water solution. Add a touch of old-fashioned sweetness by putting a few rose petals or a sprig of lavender in the vinegar. For a manly scent, use pine needles or sage.

20

Perk up a plain white sauce by adding half a teaspoon of vinegar to each cupful. Add color and zip with a sprinkling of paprika.

21

Soak hot peppers in vinegar for three or four hours and they will not burn the skin when they are cut up. And, this process seems to prevent other allergic reactions to peppers, such as dizziness.

22

If you are bothered with contact dermatitis when using most cleaning and disinfecting supplies, try pure, all natural vinegar. It cuts grease and disinfects, yet is gentle on your skin.

23

A generous splash of vinegar added to your washer's rinse cycle will fight static cling and reduce the amount of lint that settles on clothes.

24

Early vinegars did not look like the highly filtered ones familiar to today's shopper. Many of these vinegars had lots of sediment and flavorings. They were so thick they could be dehydrated and sold as sticky balls of dried vinegar. Travelers mixed these dehydrated globs with water to make "instant" vinegar.

25

Make a creamy, antioxidant fortified vinegar by combining 3/4 cup apple cider vinegar, 5 peeled garlic cloves and 1 cup each of broccoli, spinach and sweet potato in a blender. Serve over fresh greens, pasta or fruits.

26

One of the best ways to neutralize insect bites is to wipe them down with apple cider vinegar.

27

Keep a spray bottle of white vinegar in the kitchen and use it to remove lingering cooking odors from the air. It is especially useful after broiling foods or frying fish.

28

Hardboiled eggs will keep for many days if they are pickled. For a yummy variety, push 5 or 6 whole cloves into each egg. Cover the eggs with vinegar and refrigerate for several days before eating. Pepper, mustard or salt may be added to the vinegar.

29

Clean toilet bowls with a mixture of white vinegar and borax. Just wet with vinegar, sprinkle with a generous coating of borax, let stand for a couple of hours and brush away stains.

30

Add apple cider vinegar to the water meat for stews is boiled in and the meat will cook in less time and be easier to for the body to digest.

31

Soak your teapot in a strong solution of water and white vinegar to remove stains.

November

1

The added fiber in apple fortified vinegar may help remove cholesterol from the digestive system – before it can enter the blood stream and damage arteries.

2

Add a generous splash of vinegar to the water used to cook green beans and they will be less stringy, cook in less time and be easier to digest.

3

Without essential fatty acids our bodies would not function properly; cuts would not heal, hair would thin and the immune system would falter. Extra-virgin olive oil, half of the best vinaigrette, contains vitamin E and selenium. Two antioxidants that promote good health.

4

Many old home remedies for relieving muscles and tendons that become sore from overexertion use capsicin containing hot pepper vinegar as a liniment. Just pat it on and be sure to wash your hands afterwards to prevent getting it in your eyes.

5

Tangy cranberry vinegar makes a great Thanksgiving salad topper! Prepare it by gently simmering 2 cups of fresh cranberries and 2 cups of sugar in 2 cups of water until the liquid is reduced by half. Strain through a cloth and add to a quart of vinegar, along with a handful of fresh, whole berries. Great on fruit, greens or vegetables.

6

Itchy house pets will appreciate a daily vinegar rinse. Add 1/4 cup apple cider vinegar to a tub of lukewarm water and give them quick dip. It will help normalize their skin's pH balance, reducing the tendency to scratch. When scratching cannot be stopped any other way, try soaking a puppy's paws for 5 minutes a day in 3 cups water with 3 cups apple cider vinegar added to it.

7

When letting down hems, dampen them with white vinegar before pressing and it will to help remove the old creases.

8

Revitalize wilted vegetables the way Japanese cooks do – place them in a bowl of cool water with a half cup of rice vinegar added to it. In a short time the vegetables will once again be crisp and appetizing.

Old sailing ships were often out of their home ports for a year or more, making preserving food for the journey very important. One of the staple foods of these sailors was a hard, unappetizing, all-purpose biscuit made of flour and water. To make this hardtack edible they soaked it in a combination of vinegar and water to make a gruel they called skilligalee.

10

More than 125 million gallons of vinegar are produced in the United States each year. It is so important to food processors that they buy it in huge tank trucks.

11

For a sweet and creamy garlic and oil dressing, combine 1/2 cup peeled garlic cloves, 1/4 cup oil and 1/2 cup apple cider vinegar in a blender. Add 3 to 6 tablespoons of honey, depending on degree of sweetness desired. This sweet dressing is especially good on boiled potatoes or green beans.

12

Add a couple of tablespoons of vinegar to the boiling water that is used to poach eggs. The vinegar in the water will encourage the whites to remain neatly formed around the yolks, producing more appetizing, professional looking poached eggs.

13

Hundreds of years ago vinegar was a staple on sailing ships. It allowed food to be transported over great distances without rotting so it was considered the sailors' friend. They not only ate a lot of pickled foods, they used it to wash down and clean the wooden decks of ships.

14

For the very best pickled onions, always use white vinegar. It will help them retain their pale, snowy color and unique taste.

15

Vinaigrettes are a really good way to get polyunsaturated fats (like linolenic acid) from oils into the diet. Using these oils in uncooked dressings is the best way to consume them because heat can change them into trans-linoleic acid, a fat that is very unhealthy.

16

Vinegar solutions are NOT good cleaners for items made of silver. The acetic acid in it will darken, rather than brighten silver.

17

A vinaigrette of hot peppers, garlic, onion and assorted herbs makes an ideal seasoning mix for a nutritious soup. Begin with calcium fortified soup stock and add sliced onions, potatoes, carrots and other vegetables. Add 1/2 cup vinaigrette (or more to taste) and simmer until the vegetables are tender.

18

Top steamed vegetables with a low calorie dressing made by thinning 1/4 cup of fruit flavored yogurt with 1 tablespoon of apple cider vinegar. Or, use an herbal vinegar for a more intense taste.

19

Whisk together 1/2 cup rice vinegar, 1/2 cup peanut oil, 1/2 cup soy sauce, 2 cloves minced garlic and 1/4 cup honey. Use this marinade over vegetables before steaming them. This is also a great sauce for basting vegetables or meats while grilling them.

20

Turn the gravy from your Thanksgiving turkey into an exciting surprise by adding a tablespoon or so of apple cider vinegar to it. Even better, use garlic, onion, thyme or celery vinegar to perk up your gravy.

21

The acid that we know as vinegar is used by the body as a detoxifying agent. Molecules of this amazing liquid are able to connect themselves to many dangerous substances, including some drugs and poisons. This action creates entirely new compounds, which tend to be biologically inactive. Then, these harmless substances can be safely expelled by the body.

22

Leavening is the process that lightens both dough and batters. Tiny bubbles of moist air form and then expand during cooking to make foods lighter. Vinegar causes this when it reacts with baking soda. During baking carbon dioxide is released in the form of moist air pockets. Then, these tiny bubbles slowly expand, adding to the lightness of the food.

23

Both migraines and tension headaches increase when magnesium levels are low. Apple cider vinegar supplies this important mineral.

24

One reason that dieters often combine vinegar with mustard or cayenne pepper is that they each burn more calories than they contain. This is because both mustard and cayenne boost the metabolic rate. Each quarter of an ounce can cause the body to use up as much as 60 extra calories!

25

In the United States, retail sales account for 24% of vinegar use, the manufacture of pickles for 20%. The other 56% is used to make salad dressings, mayonnaise, catsup, mustard and other vinegar-based food products.

26

Simply inhaling the delightful aroma of vaporized vinegar can kill flu germs. This makes it a good choice when fighting a cold.

27

When preparing a pot roast, be sure to add a generous splash of vinegar to the pot. It will make the meat more tender and easier to digest.

28

Preserved pickles that are not completely covered with liquid MUST be disposed of without tasting! Cucumbers not covered with vinegar can cause severe food poisoning, even death.

29

Deter mold from forming on cheese by wrapping it in a cloth dampened with white vinegar. Put the cloth-wrapped cheese in a plastic bag and store it in the refrigerator.

30

Natural, organic, unfiltered vinegar will contain fine particles of the food used to make it. A sediment at the bottom of the bottle is the sign of a high quality, unfiltered vinegar.

December

1

Fermentation, such as the process that changes fresh, perishable foods into long lasting vinegar, transforms food particles into smaller molecules. Another example of fermentation is when yeast ferments the complex sugar, glucose, into less complex substances. Because this makes food more digestible some cultures call fermented foods 'predigested foods.'

2

Add creases to pant legs, especially those made of knit fabrics, by dampening the fabric with white vinegar before ironing them. This is also a good way to renew old creases in any fabric.

3

Add a tablespoon or two of apple cider vinegar to a pot of baked beans and they will be easier to digest.

4

Make herbal vinegars especially pleasing to the eye by placing a sprig of fresh herb in the bottle. Or, add a few ripe berries to berry vinegars. These pretty liquids make great gifts for family and friends!

5

Make a clear vinaigrette by combining 1/2 apple cider vinegar and 1/2 cup oil. This is a simple, uncomplicated dressing that does not overwhelm delicate vegetables like asparagus.

6

Balsamic vinegar is a great topping for fresh or lightly blanched vegetables; no need to add oil or spices.

7

The oldest commercial production method (named after the French city where it originated in the 1600s) is the Orleans, or slow process. Using this method, a single batch of vinegar takes from 4 to 12 weeks to complete.

8

Cauliflower that is going to be used with vegetable dips will stay snowy white longer if it is first rinsed in a mixture of 1 quart water and 1/4 cup white vinegar.

9

Stainless steel will gleam like new when wiped down with full-strength white vinegar. You can polish the metal dry with a soft cloth, without rinsing the vinegar off.

10

Thin yogurt, plain or fruit flavored, with a small amount of apple cider vinegar for a healthful dressing for fruit salads.

11

For a healthy vinegar dressing, put 1/2 cup apple cider vinegar, 1/2 cup sunflower oil, 1 cup spinach, 1 cup celery, 1 green bell pepper, 1 large carrot and 1 teaspoon basil into a blender. Mix until smooth and add to a leafy salad or boiled pasta. Or, for a special treat, drizzle this healthy green dressing generously over cubes of cold meat. It contains vitamin C and zinc to help you resist colds and thiamin, riboflavin and vitamin B-6 to discourage depression.

12

Replace sour milk or buttermilk in recipes by putting 1 1/2 teaspoons of vinegar in a glass measuring cup and filling it with milk. Stir after 3 minutes and it will be ready to use.

13

One of the best ways to use your own homemade vinegars is to put them in pretty decanters with shaker tops. Keep an assortment on the table to replace the salt shaker.

14

Make an especially tasty meat sauce by mixing pan drippings with an equal amount of garlic vinegar. Dilute with water for a milder tasting topping; add a tiny splash of hot pepper vinegar for a zippier tasting topping.

15

Apple cider vinegar may be substituted for rice vinegar in recipes by adding 1/2 cup water to each pint of the apple cider vinegar. This weakened apple cider vinegar will taste and react in recipes very much like the milder, less acidic rice vinegar.

16

Add a little vinegar to egg based cooked sauces and they will be less likely to curdle. This works because vinegar helps keep eggs suspended in sauces, thereby raising the temperature at which their protein turns into a solid. Plain egg protein coagulates at 160°F, when vinegar is added it rises to 195°F, permitting you to cook the sauce more thoroughly before the egg congeals.

17

Pickle lovers who need to avoid salt can make their own healthy alternative. Simple add a pre-mixed packet of pickling spice to a quart of warm apple cider vinegar, add cucumbers and age for a couple of weeks. Or, you can mix up your own favorite pickling spices in a bottle of apple cider vinegar.

18

Mustard is a digestive stimulant. Use it and vinegar together for their health benefits, their great taste and for their low calorie ability to stimulate the digestive process. Make salt free mustard by blending dry mustard and vinegar together until they are the consistency of thick batter. Then add a few drops of oil. This is a good sauce for rubbing down meats before they are grilled.

19

France has been famous since the 1500s for producing excellent truffles, a subterranean fungus that was thought to be an aphrodisiac. One of the most popular ways to serve and preserve them was pickled in vinegar. To serve them, they are pulled out of the vinegar, soaked briefly in hot water and served with lots of fresh butter.

20

Creamy vinegars can add significant amounts of beta-carotene and vegetable flavorids to food. These antioxidants help the body repair the damage done by free radicals. Clear vinegars leach vitamins, minerals and trace elements from herbs soaked in it.

21

The people of old Pompeii preserved onions in a mixture of vinegar and salt. Pickled onions are still considered a delicious treat.

22

When butter was first commercially produced, a small amount of vinegar was used on the butter wrappers to inhibit mold growth. It protected the butter without adding harsh or poisonous chemicals

23

Vinegar is a low salt, low calorie, no cholesterol seasoning! It is a way to enhance flavors, and bring new ones to the table, without adding undesirable additives and calories. Almost any bland food can be enlivened with a splash or two of vinegar.

24

Remove wine stains by dampening them with white vinegar, then blotting the stain away.

25

Use warm fennel vinegar as a facial astringent. It will clean pores and condition the skin. As an added bonus, its hormone-like action fights wrinkles.

26

Soak tough stewing chicken for an hour in a mixture of 3/4 cup vinegar, 1/2 cup oil and 1 thinly sliced lemon. Drain and cook as if it were a young fryer.

27

Listeria is a bacteria found on nearly 20% of all hot dogs. The illness it causes is especially dangerous to babies and the elderly. Neutralize this bacteria by boiling hot dogs for a few minutes in water with a couple of tablespoons of apple cider vinegar added to it.

28

Umeboshi plums are a sour, heavily salted food that Traditional Chinese Medicine considers medicinal. These plums are pickled in cedar vats for several weeks to draw out their natural juices. They are then dried in the sun before being put back in the juice with plant leaves that turn them a dark pink color. Often, they are aged for a year or more before being served.

29

A dash of white vinegar in the cooking water makes for snow-white mashed potatoes. This is also effective when boiling cauliflower.

30

Béarnaise sauce is a classic topping for broiled fish. Prepare it by gently simmering together for one minute, 1 cup white wine, 2 tablespoons white wine vinegar and 1 tablespoon minced onion. Whisk 1/2 cup soft butter and 3 egg yolks into this mixture and heat until it begins to thicken; do not boil. Season the finished sauce with a teaspoon each of tarragon, parsley and chervil. Serve with a sprinkling of cayenne and white peppers. (Leeks or shallots may be used in place of onions.)

31

Cinnamon and cloves are two of the many spices that magnify vinegar's power to curb bacterial growth. Nutmeg and allspice are less effective but also of some help in the preservation of food.

Questions and Answers

Question: I have diabetes, a heart condition, arthritis, etc. Is it safe for me to take vinegar every day?

Answer: If you have a chronic medical condition ALWAYS check with a health care professional before adding anything, including vinegar, to your diet.

Question: I take medication. Can vinegar be taken with it?

Answer: If you take medication, including over the counter drugs, ALWAYS check with a health care professional before adding vinegar to your diet.

Question: Will vinegar pull calcium from my bones?

Answer: No. Vinegar in the digestive system does not come into direct contact with your bones. It works in other ways to aid health.

Question: What kind of vinegar should I use?

Answer: Use white vinegar for cleaning and to pickle light colored foods. Use apple cider vinegar for tonics and most recipes. Rice, champagne, wine and other vinegars can also be used in recipes.

Question: Where can I find herbal vinegars?

Answer: More and more supermarkets now carry a line of herbal vinegars. For the freshest, most robust flavor make your own by adding a few tablespoons of an herb to a good supermarket vinegar.

Question: Where can I find organic vinegar?

Answer: A few supermarkets now carry organic vinegar, as do many health food stores. Some mail order specialty houses sell organic vinegar, too.

Preferred Customer Reorder Form

Order this...	If you want a book on...	Cost...	Number of Copies...
Amish Gardening Secrets	You too can learn the special gardening secrets the Amish use to produce huge tomato plants and bountiful harvests. Information packed 800-plus collection for you to tinker with and enjoy.	$9.95	
Home Remedies from the Old South	Hundreds of little known old-time remedies for aches & pains, cleaning & beauty.	$9.95	
The Vinegar Home Guide	Learn how to clean and freshen with natural, environmentally-safe vinegar in the house, garden and laundry. Plus, delicious home-style recipes!	$9.95	
Emily's Disaster Guide of Natural Remedies	Emily's new guide to infectious diseases & their threat on our health. What happens if we can't get to the pharmacy – or the shelves are empty, *what then?* What if the electricity goes out – and stays out? What if my neighborhood was quarantined? How would I feed my family? Handle first aid? 208 page book!	$9.95	

Any combination of the above $9.95 items qualifies for the following discounts...

| | | **Total NUMBER of $9.95 items** | |

Order any 2 items for: $15.95	Order any 4 items for: $24.95	Order any 6 items for: $34.95	Any additional items for: $5 each
Order any 3 items for: $19.95	Order any 5 items for: $29.95	**and receive 7th item FREE**	

FEATURED SELECTIONS		Total COST of $9.95 items	
The Vinegar Anniversary Book	Completely updated with the latest research and brand new remedies and uses for apple cider vinegar. Handsome coffee table collector's edition you'll be proud to display. ***Big 208-page book!***	$12.95	
The Magic of Baking Soda	*Plain Old Baking Soda A Drugstore in A Box?* Doctors & researchers have discovered baking soda has amazing healing properties! Over 600 health & Household Hints. *Great Recipes Too!*	$12.95	
Vinegar Formula Guide	This one-of-a-kind, ground breaking book gives you exact formulas and measurements for ALL of your vinegar applications! In it you'll find step-by-step, easy-to-use instructions for home health remedies, cleaning projects and more!	$19.95	
The Cinnamon Book	Research studies have found this amazing spice is loaded with health benefits. Find out how cinnamon can be used in treating common (and not so common) conditions such as diabetes, obesity, arthritis, high cholesterol and a host of other ailments.	$19.95	
The Magic of Hydrogen Peroxide	An Ounce of Hydrogen Peroxide is worth a Pound of Cure! Hundreds of health cures, household uses & home remedy uses for hydrogen peroxide contained in this breakthrough volume.	$19.95	

Order any 2 or more Featured Selections for only $10 each...

	Postage & Handling	$3.98*
	TOTAL	

90-Day Money-Back Guarantee

* Shipping of 10 or more books = $6.96

Please rush me the items marked above. I understand that I must be completely satisfied or I can return any item within 90 days with proof of purchase for a full and prompt refund of my purchase price.

I am enclosing $_____ by: ❏ Check ❏ Money Order (Make checks payable to James Direct Inc)

Charge my credit card Signature _____

Card No. _____ Exp. Date _____

Name _____ Address _____

City _____ State _____ Zip _____

Telephone Number (_____) _____

❏ Yes! I'd like to know about freebies, specials and new products before they are nationally advertised. My email address is: _____

Mail To: **James Direct Inc.** • PO Box 980, Dept. A1229 • Hartville, Ohio 44632
Customer Service (330) 877-0800 • *http://www.jamesdirect.com*

©2013 JDI A216IM

AMISH GARDENING SECRETS

There's something for everyone in *Amish Gardening Secrets*. This BIG collection contains over 800 gardening hints, suggestions, time savers and tonics that have been passed down over the years in Amish communities and elsewhere.

- -

HOME REMEDIES FROM THE OLD SOUTH

Emily Thacker's original collection of old-time remedies. Hundreds of little-known cures from yesteryear on how to lose weight, beautify skin, help arthritis. A collection of more than 700 remedies Grandma used for colds, sinus, sexual dysfunction, gout, hangovers, asthma, urinary infections, headaches, and appetite control.

- -

THE VINEGAR HOME GUIDE

Emily Thacker presents her second volume of hundreds of all-new vinegar tips. Use versatile vinegar to add a low-sodium zap of flavor to your cooking, as well as getting your house "white-glove" clean for just pennies. Plus, safe and easy tips on shining and polishing brass, copper & pewter and removing stubborn stains & static cling in your laundry!

- -

EMILY'S DISASTER GUIDE OF NATURAL REMEDIES

Emily's most important book yet! If large groups of the population become sick at the same time, the medical services in this country will become stressed to capacity. *What then*? We will all need to know what to do! Over 307 natural cures, preventatives, cure-alls and ways to prepare to naturally treat & prevent infectious disease.

- -

THE VINEGAR ANNIVERSARY BOOK

Handsome coffee table edition and brand new information on Mother Nature's Secret Weapon – apple cider vinegar!

- -

THE MAGIC OF BAKING SODA

We all know baking soda works like magic around the house. It cleans, deodorizes & works wonders in the kitchen and in the garden. But did you know it's an effective remedy for allergies, bladder infection, heart disorders... *and MORE!*

NEW
- -

VINEGAR FORMULA GUIDE

Studies have shown vinegar to be effective at not only cleaning and disinfecting, but also as a natural home remedy for conditions such as lowering cholesterol, fighting disease, easing arthritis, improving circulation and more! Now learn the exact formulas and measurements for EACH home remedy and cleaning project in a concise, easy-to-read format! No more guesswork!

NEW
- -

THE CINNAMON BOOK

Cinnamon is rich in natural healing properties such as being an anti-oxidant, anti-inflammatory, anti-coagulant, anti-microbial, anti-parasitic, anti-tumor – just to name a few! Find out how cinnamon can be used to fight everything from simple cuts and scrapes to chronic health condition, safely and naturally!

- -

THE MAGIC OF HYDROGEN PEROXIDE

Hundreds of health cures & home remedy uses for hydrogen peroxide. You'll be amazed to see how a little hydrogen peroxide mixed with a pinch of this or that from your cupboard can do everything from relieving chronic pain to making age spots go away! Easy household cleaning formulas too!

* Each Book has its own FREE Bonus!

Preferred Customer Reorder Form

Order this...	If you want a book on...	Cost...	Number of Copies...
Amish Gardening Secrets	You too can learn the special gardening secrets the Amish use to produce huge tomato plants and bountiful harvests. Information packed 800-plus collection for you to tinker with and enjoy.	$9.95	
Home Remedies from the Old South	Hundreds of little known old-time remedies for aches & pains, cleaning & beauty.	$9.95	
The Vinegar Home Guide	Learn how to clean and freshen with natural, environmentally-safe vinegar in the house, garden and laundry. Plus, delicious home-style recipes!	$9.95	
Emily's Disaster Guide of Natural Remedies	Emily's new guide to infectious diseases & their threat on our health. What happens if we can't get to the pharmacy – or the shelves are empty, *what then?* What if the electricity goes out – and stays out? What if my neighborhood was quarantined? How would I feed my family? Handle first aid? 208 page book!	$9.95	

Any combination of the above $9.95 items qualifies for the following discounts...

Total NUMBER of $9.95 items	

Order any 2 items for: $15.95

Order any 3 items for: $19.95

Order any 4 items for: $24.95

Order any 5 items for: $29.95

Order any 6 items for: $34.95 **and receive 7th item FREE**

Any additional items for: $5 each

FEATURED SELECTIONS		Total COST of $9.95 items	
The Vinegar Anniversary Book	Completely updated with the latest research and brand new remedies and uses for apple cider vinegar. Handsome coffee table collector's edition you'll be proud to display. ***Big 208-page book!***	$12.95	
The Magic of Baking Soda	*Plain Old Baking Soda A Drugstore in A Box?* Doctors & researchers have discovered baking soda has amazing healing properties! Over 600 health & Household Hints. *Great Recipes Too!*	$12.95	
Vinegar Formula Guide	This one-of-a-kind, ground breaking book gives you exact formulas and measurements for ALL of your vinegar applications! In it you'll find step-by-step, easy-to-use instructions for home health remedies, cleaning projects and more!	$19.95	
The Cinnamon Book	Research studies have found this amazing spice is loaded with health benefits. Find out how cinnamon can be used in treating common (and not so common) conditions such as diabetes, obesity, arthritis, high cholesterol and a host of other ailments.	$19.95	
The Magic of Hydrogen Peroxide	An Ounce of Hydrogen Peroxide is worth a Pound of Cure! Hundreds of health cures, household uses & home remedy uses for hydrogen peroxide contained in this breakthrough volume.	$19.95	

Order any 2 or more Featured Selections for only $10 each...

Postage & Handling	$3.98*
TOTAL	

*** Shipping of 10 or more books = $6.96**

90-DAY MONEY-BACK GUARANTEE

Please rush me the items marked above. I understand that I must be completely satisfied or I can return any item within 90 days with proof of purchase for a full and prompt refund of my purchase price.

I am enclosing $_____ by: ❑ Check ❑ Money Order (Make checks payable to James Direct Inc)

Charge my credit card Signature _____

Card No. _____ Exp. Date _____

Name _____ Address _____

City _____ State _____ Zip _____

Telephone Number (_____) _____

❑ Yes! I'd like to know about freebies, specials and new products before they are nationally advertised. My email address is: _____

Mail To: **James Direct Inc.** • PO Box 980, Dept. A1229 • Hartville, Ohio 44632
Customer Service (330) 877-0800 • *http://www.jamesdirect.com*

©2013 JDI A216IM

AMISH GARDENING SECRETS

There's something for everyone in *Amish Gardening Secrets*. This BIG collection contains over 800 gardening hints, suggestions, time savers and tonics that have been passed down over the years in Amish communities and elsewhere.

- -

HOME REMEDIES FROM THE OLD SOUTH

Emily Thacker's original collection of old-time remedies. Hundreds of little-known cures from yesteryear on how to lose weight, beautify skin, help arthritis. A collection of more than 700 remedies Grandma used for colds, sinus, sexual dysfunction, gout, hangovers, asthma, urinary infections, headaches, and appetite control.

- -

THE VINEGAR HOME GUIDE

Emily Thacker presents her second volume of hundreds of all-new vinegar tips. Use versatile vinegar to add a low-sodium zap of flavor to your cooking, as well as getting you house "white-glove" clean for just pennies. Plus, safe and easy tips on shining and polishing brass, copper & pewter and removing stubborn stains & static cling in your laundry!

- -

EMILY'S DISASTER GUIDE OF NATURAL REMEDIES

Emily's most important book yet! If large groups of the population become sick at the same time, the medical services in this country will become stressed to capacity. *What then* We will all need to know what to do! Over 307 natural cures, preventatives, cure-alls and ways to prepare to naturally treat & prevent infectious disease.

- -

THE VINEGAR ANNIVERSARY BOOK

Handsome coffee table edition and brand new information on Mother Nature's Secret Weapon – apple cider vinegar!

- -

THE MAGIC OF BAKING SODA

We all know baking soda works like magic around the house. It cleans, deodorizes & works wonders in the kitchen and in the garden. But did you know it's an effective remedy for allergies, bladder infection, heart disorders… *and MORE!*

NEW -

VINEGAR FORMULA GUIDE

Studies have shown vinegar to be effective at not only cleaning and disinfecting, but also as a natural home remedy for conditions such as lowering cholesterol, fighting disease, easing arthritis, improving circulation and more! Now learn the exact formulas and measurements for EACH home remedy and cleaning project in a concise, easy-to-read format! No more guesswork!

NEW -

THE CINNAMON BOOK

Cinnamon is rich in natural healing properties such as being an anti-oxidant, anti-inflammatory, anti-coagulant, anti-microbial, anti-parasitic, anti-tumor – just to name a few Find out how cinnamon can be used to fight everything from simple cuts and scrapes to chronic health condition, safely and naturally!

- -

THE MAGIC OF HYDROGEN PEROXIDE

Hundreds of health cures & home remedy uses for hydrogen peroxide. You'll be amazed to see how a little hydrogen peroxide mixed with a pinch of this or that from your cupboard can do everything from relieving chronic pain to making age spots go away! Easy household cleaning formulas too!

* Each Book has its own FREE Bonus!

> All these important books carry our NO-RISK GUARANTEE. Enjoy them for three full months. If you are not 100% satisfied simply return the book(s) along with proof of purchase, for a prompt, "no questions asked" refund!

Index

You will notice that *vinegar* is not listed in the index. That is because the word vinegar is on virtually every page of the book.